THE POST-SURGICAL PAIN DIARY

Tracking Your Pain,
Progress & Physical Therapy
after Surgery

THE POST-SURGICAL PAIN DIARY

Tracking Your Pain,
Progress & Physical Therapy
after Surgery

The Post-Surgical Pain Diary: Tracking Your Pain, Progress & Physical Therapy after Surgery

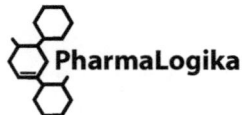

Author: Mindy J. Allport-Settle

Published by PharmaLogika, Inc.

Printed in the United States of America.

ISBN-13 978-1-937258-04-7

Acknowledgements

While many people helped make this book possible, useful and successful, special thanks go to:

Judy A. McComb, MBA

Linda A. Holliday, MEd

Jeanne McComb

and

Elisabeth Johnson, RN, NP

CONTENTS

Acknowledgements v

Overview 1

    About this Book 1

        Included Documents and Features 1

Introduction 3

    Instructions for Using this Book 3

Examples 5

Medical History 17

Monthly Summaries 27

Daily Summaries 33

About this Book

After surgery, it is essential to track your level of pain and your progress through physical therapy. Receiving appropriate treatment for any medical condition requires providing complete and accurate information to your medical team. Often, it will require more than one visit to more than one medical professional. Each visit requires completing similar forms and each of those professionals will likely ask many of the same questions, but with a slightly different focus.

This book has been designed and tested to help keep track of the frequently long and arduous process of healing after surgery and successfully managing pain. The needs of the patient, the clinician, and the many supportive members of the medical team (including the patient's family) are balanced to provide an easy reference tool with precise results. The included forms are modeled on the principles of good clinical practices and patient questionnaire requirements for clinical study protocols.

Each page provides a graphical snapshot of critical data and factors related to the many causes of pain, trends over time and treatment effectiveness. It is an invaluable communication tool between the patient and medical team that leads to faster solutions for effective treatment and better treatment compliance for the patient. Additionally, sections are provided for you to record some general medical history information to make certain you have everything in one place when you need it.

Included Documents and Features

- Examples for completing each set of data records

- Comprehensive personal and family medical history section detailing health conditions and possible inherited traits

- Monthly data summaries for easy long term trend analysis

- Daily data records condensing critical information for diagnostic and treatment evaluation and trend analysis

Pain is to be expected after surgery and it is a completely normal part of the post-surgery healing process. The ability to recognize problems after surgery and the success of your treatment plan both rely on your ability to accurately report information to your medical team. You are your own best advocate and this book will provide you with the best tool for collaborating with your medical team.

Pain is a *part* of you, but it is not *you*. It is not who you are. It does not define you. It can, however, dictate the choices you make every day. Your physical therapy following surgery will be strenuous and, at times, uncomfortable. It will help you overcome your pain given commitment, patience, and time.

As difficult as pain is to live with, pain is also a useful tool. It lets us know when there is a problem with a part of our body that we need to treat. It also lets us know when we are healing, building new and stronger muscle tissue, and when we have pushed too far or too hard in our efforts to heal. The type and level of pain you experience creates a map detailing whether your healing process is moving forward as expected or if you need to adjust your treatment plan.

This book is designed to provide a map of the path your pain takes as well as a means to track the effects of the treatments you use. It will provide your medical team with a comprehensive and concise tool to monitor your response to different treatments and triggers over time so they can best assist you in the management of your pain. By documenting your progress, you will be able to manage your pain more effectively.

Instructions for Using this Book

While it looks like an overwhelming amount of information to document every day, keep in mind that this is meant to be a short term tool designed to help solve what could otherwise become a long term problem. This book will make your life, and your medical team's job, easier.

Answer the questions and complete the charts that apply to you. Work with your medical team to determine which tools in the book will help them develop the best treatment plan for you. Typically, just a couple of weeks worth of data will be invaluable in determining if your pain is decreasing as expected. Additionally, this book should be used as you start new treaments to document how you respond to each form of treatment and quickly steer you toward the best options.

There are two critical directions to keep in mind about this book:

1.) ***Do not become addicted*** to writing in this book and chronicling every second of your day. Focusing that much on the quantity and quality of your pain can increase the intensity and duration of the pain you experience.

2.) ***Do not become overwhelmed*** by the number of pages and the amount of information requested in this book. Only fill out the sections that are important to you. Remember that this book is just a tool for you to use in communicating with your medical team.

When you are in pain it is difficult to remember each aspect of your medical history – but it is the time you need it the most.

The pages in this book are designed to collect comprehensive information. They provide a unique hourly and daily graphical view of your pain scale with exact locations, therapeutic treatments, sleep patterns, exercise and activity levels, physical therapy regimens, physiological patterns and changes, and specific drug reactions.

Based on the criteria developed for clinical drug and medical device trials, this graphical interface design documents your pain in a way that is familiar to your medical team so they can quickly recognize patterns and devise an effective treatment plan that will adequately treat your pain.

The following section provides examples of how each page should be completed by you. Take this book with you to your medical appointments so you can discuss the tracked data with your medical team. They might choose to photocopy some of the pages so they can include the tracked data in your chart for later review.

1 DAILY TREATMENT PLAN

As you and your medical team develop new treatment plans, record your plan for the day including:
1) New medications,
2) Increases or decreases to medications,
3) Exercises, physical therapy, or any other treatments,
4) It will be especially helpful to record any side effects you experience as you add new treatments. This can help determine which types of treatments will work best for you.

Contact your care provider with any bad reactions or side effects to determine if you should the medication or treatment.

MEDICATION / TREATMENT	AMOUNT / TIME / COMMENTS
Gabapentin	Increase to 600 mg twice today
Tramadol	Decrease to 50 mg in the morning onl
Alprazolam	Take right before going to bed → felt
Stretching	
Stationary Bike	
Physical Therapy	

5 DAILY PAIN SUMMARY

Were there times during the day that you experienced unrelieved breakthrough pain? ___NO ✓YES

How many times did this happen today?

1 2 3 ④ 5 6 7 8 9 10 more than 10

Did any specific activity start your breakthrough pain?
___NO ✓YES: What activities?
Bending Over

Put an "X" on the body diagram to show each place you've had BREAKTHROUGH PAIN today.

What was your average level of pain today?

0 1 2 3 4 ⑤ 6 7 8 9 10

Other than prescription medicine, did you do anything else today to relieve the pain? ___NO ✓YES:
(Note any that you used.)
✓ Non-prescription drugs (e.g., acetaminophen, ibuprofen)
___ Herbal remedies
✓ Hot or cold packs
✓ Exercise
✓ Changing position (such as lying down or elevating your legs)
___ Physical therapy
___ Massage
___ Acupuncture
✓ Rest
___ Prayer, meditation, guided imagery
___ Relaxation technique (hypnosis, biofeedback)
___ Creative technique (art or music therapy)
✓ Other (e.g., specific chiropractic manipulation, osteopathic treatments):
_____

Check any of these common side effects that you've noticed after taking your pain medicine:
___ Drowsiness, sleepiness
___ Nausea, vomiting, upset stomach

6 DAILY BODY PAIN DIAGRAM

Mark each place on the diagram where you have had pain today by placing an 'X', circling the location, or shading the area.

Describe the type of pain:

Shooting   Deep
Tingling   Sharp
Numbness   Burning / Hot
Cold   Aching
Surface Pain   Gnawing / Biting
Stabbing   Electrical / Shocks
Dull   Other _____
Stinging

Your Right Side

Sharp

Tingling

Sharp

Front

2 DAILY PAIN CHART

DAY Monday DATE Sept. 26, 2011 WEIGHT 223

INSTRUCTIONS:
1.) Place an 'X' on the chart below where the lines for the time of day and your level of pain meet.
2.) Connect the points on your DAILY PAIN CHART so your medical team can see when your status changed.
3.) Refer to the EXAMPLES in the front of this book for further direction.

PAIN LEVEL
WORST IMAGINABLE 10
9
8
7
6
MODERATE 5
4
3
2
1
NONE 0

3 DAILY MEDICATION

MEDICINE NAME / DOSE
1 Neurontin (600mg)
2 Tramadol (50mg)
3 All regular pills
4
5
6
7
8
9

4 DAILY PHYSIOLOGY

SLEEP
RESTROOM
NAUSEA / DIZZINESS
MEAL / SNACK
EXERCISE / PHYSICAL THERAPY
STRESS / ANXIETY Physical Therapy

	BLOOD PRESSURE	PULSE
	180 / 86	78
	152 / 78	92

EXAMPLES

1 PERSONAL
MEDICAL TEAM SUMMARY

NAME	PHONE	FAX	NOTES
Dr. John Smith	919-555-1212	919-557-6789	Primary Care Physician
ADDRESS			Kathy, Nurse
Family Practice			
123 North Judd Parkway NE			
Fuquay-Varina, NC 27526			

NAME	PHONE	FAX	NOTES
Dr. Jill Murphy			OB-Gyn
ADDRESS			Option 5 for Nurse
Women's Health			
Raleigh, NC			

NAME	PHONE	FAX	NOTES
Dr. David Thomas	919-782-3456		Neurologist
ADDRESS			Medical Record #
Neurology Clinic			41283367
1540 Abizaid Drive			
Raleigh, NC			

NAME	PHONE	FAX	NOTES
ADDRESS			

NAME	PHONE	FAX	NOTES
ADDRESS			

2 CURRENT PERSCRIPTION MEDICATIONS

DRUG NAME	DOSAGE	FREQUENCY	TREATMENT FOR	SIDE EFFECTS
Gabapentin	600 mg	2 / day	Neuropathy	Drowsiness
Lisinopril	20 mg	1 / day	High Blood Pressure	None
Tramadol	50 mg	1 / day	Pain	Constipation
Fluoxetine	10 mg	1 / day	Depression	Nausea
Alprazolam	0.5 mg	as needed	Anxiety	Drowsiness

3 CURRENT OVER THE COUNTER MEDICATIONS (ASPIRIN, ETC.)

DRUG NAME	DOSAGE	FREQUENCY	TREATMENT FOR	SIDE EFFECTS
Allegra-D		2 / day	Allergies	

4 DRUG ALLERGY SUMMARY

DRUG NAME (include prescription and other medicines)	REACTION
Erythromycin	Extreme Nausea
Rocephin	Hives, Itching

5 PAIN SURVEY

Place a check (✓) in the appropriate box.

ACTIVITY	None	Mild	Moderate	Severe	Unable	HELPFUL TREATMENTS / COMMENTS
Pain when performing the following?						
Bending				✓		
Caring for Infirm Family	✓					N/A
Carrying Groceries		✓				
Changing Position (Sit to Stand)			✓			
Climbing Stairs			✓			
Driving		✓				
Extended Computer Use			✓			
Feeding (Self)		✓				
Household Chores			✓			
Kneeling		✓				
Lifting Children			✓			
Lifting objects			✓			
Pet Care		✓				
Reading (Concentration)	✓					
Self care - Bathing			✓			
Self care - Dressing			✓			
Self care - Shaving			✓			
Sexual Activities				✓		
Sleeping		✓				Ibuprofen & Heating Pad
Sitting (Prolonged)			✓			
Standing (Prolonged)			✓			
Walking			✓			
Yard Work				✓		
Sports / Recreational Activities / Exercise				✓		
List:						
List:						
List:						
List:						
List:						
List any other activities that cause pain:						

MEDICAL HISTORY EXAMPLES

6 PERSONAL & FAMILY
HEALTH HISTORY (PAGE 1 OF 3)

Place a check (✓) in the corresponding box for each condition as it applies to you and you relatives.

Condition	You	Your Mother	Your Father	Brother(s)	Sister(s)	Maternal Grandmother	Maternal Grandfather	Maternal Aunt(s)/Uncle(s)	Paternal Grandmother	Paternal Grandfather	Paternal Aunt(s)/Uncle(s)	Comments
Head (Ear, Nose, Throat / Eyes / Jaw):												
Migraine Headaches												
Severe / Frequent Headaches	X											
Jaw Pain / TMJ	X	X				X						
Dizziness or Faintness												
Epilepsy / Seizures or Convulsions												
Near or Farsighted (Glasses)	X	X			X	X	X		X		X	
Glaucoma												
Cataracts												
Blindness												
Recurrent Ear Infecitons												
Deafness / Reduced Hearing						X						
Hay Fever	X	X										
Recurrent Sinusitis												
Overactive Thyroid (Hyperthyroidism)												
Underactive Thyroid (Hypothyroidism)	X						X					
Goiter												
Other:_____												
Psychological:												
Smoking	X											Quit at 35
Alcoholism			X				X					
Chemical Dependency												
Anxiety							X					
Serious Depression												
Post Traumatic Stress Disorder (PTSD)												
Nervous Breakdown												
Suicide / Attempt			X									
Bipolar Disorder				X								
Personality Disorder:_____												
Neurological (Nerves):												
Insomnia	X	X	X	X	X	X	X	X				
Sleep Apnea							X					
Peripheral Neuropathy	X					X						
Paralysis												
Orthopedic (Bones, Muscles, etc.):												
Arthritis / Swollen Joints / Rheumatism		X				X	X					
Osteoporosis												
Varicose Veins		X				X						
Connective Tissue Disorder												
Gout												
Broken Bones	X						X					
Cortisone Treatments												
Artificial Joints												
Swollen Feet or Ankles						X	X					
Back Problems / Injury			X									

7 MEDICATION SIDE EFFECTS

As you and your medical team develop new treatment plans, it will be especially helpful to record any side effects you experience as you add new treatments. This can help determine which types of treatments will work best for you.

Contact your care provider with any side effects.

MEDICATION NAME	DATE STARTED	DATE STOPPED	SIDE EFFECTS / COMMENTS
Gabapentin	2009		Drowsiness
Lisinopril	2010		None
Tramadol	2009	Sept 2011	Constipation
Fluoxetine	Feb 2011		Nausea at 20 mg, dropped to 10 mg
Alprazolam	Sept 2011		Drowsiness ⟶ XR felt too drugged
Allegra-D	2005		None / Only take in Spring & Fall
Erythromycin	1992	1992	ALLERGIC / Extreme Nausea
Rocephin	June 2011	June 2011	ALLERGIC / Hives, Itching

MEDICAL HISTORY EXAMPLES

1 DAILY
TREATMENT PLAN

As you and your medical team develop new treatment plans, record your plan for the day including:
1.) New medications,
2.) Increases or decreases to medications,
3.) Exercises, physical therapy, or any other treatments,
4.) It will be especially helpful to record any side effects you experience as you add new treatments.
   This can help determine which types of treatments will work best for you.

Contact your care provider with any bad reactions or side effects to determine if you should discontinue the medication or treatment.

MEDICATION / TREATMENT	AMOUNT / TIME / COMMENTS
Gabapentin	Increase to 600 mg twice today
Tramadol	Decrease to 50 mg in the morning only
Alprazolam	Take right before going to bed → felt too drugged
Stretching	Increase to twice today
Stationary Bike	Increase to twice today
Physical Therapy	Meet at 3pm

DAY __Monday__ DATE __Sept. 26, 2011__ WEIGHT __223__

INSTRUCTIONS:
1.) **Place an 'X'** on the chart below where the lines for the time of day and your level of pain meet.
2.) **Connect the points** on your DAILY PAIN CHART so your medical team can see when your status changed.
3.) **Refer to the EXAMPLES** in the front of this book for further direction.

2 DAILY PAIN CHART

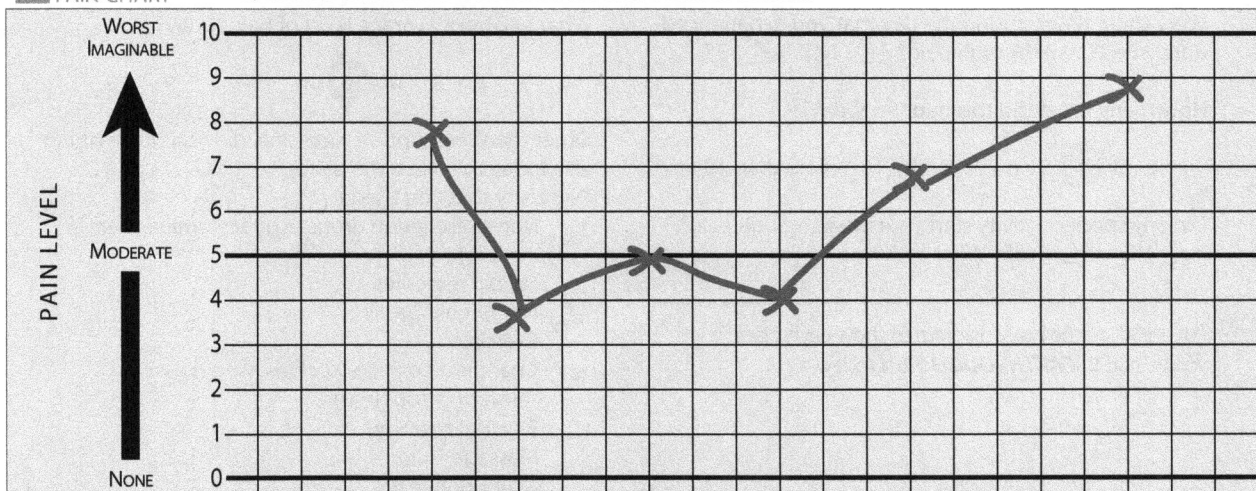

PAIN LEVEL

WORST IMAGINABLE — 10
9
8
7
MODERATE — 5
4
3
2
1
NONE — 0

3 DAILY MEDICATION

MEDICINE NAME / DOSE

	Medicine	
1	Neurontin (600mg)	
2	Tramadol (50mg)	
3	All regular pills	
4		
5		
6		
7		
8		
9		

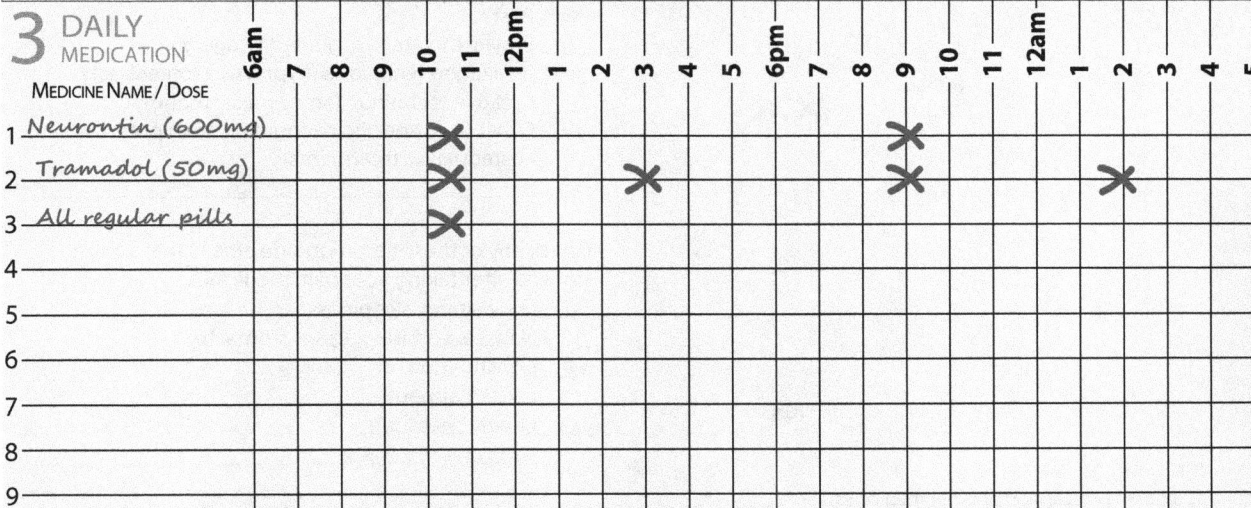

4 DAILY PHYSIOLOGY

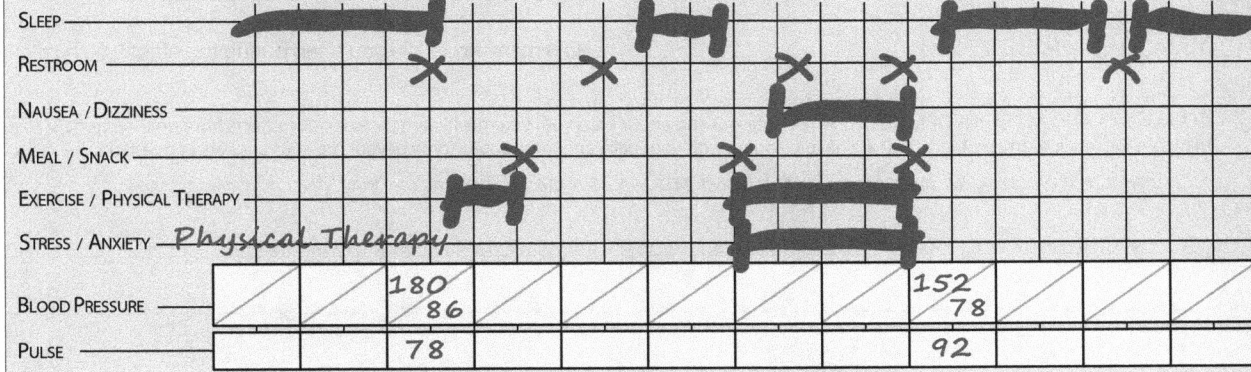

SLEEP
RESTROOM
NAUSEA / DIZZINESS
MEAL / SNACK
EXERCISE / PHYSICAL THERAPY
STRESS / ANXIETY — Physical Therapy

BLOOD PRESSURE — 180/86 ... 152/78

PULSE — 78 ... 92

5 DAILY
PAIN SUMMARY

Were there times during the day that you experienced unrelieved breakthrough pain? _____NO ✓YES

How many times did this happen today?

1 2 3 ④ 5 6 7 8 9 10   more than 10

Did any specific activity start your breakthrough pain? _____NO ✓YES: What activities?

Bending Over

Put an "X" on the body diagram to show each place you've had **BREAKTHROUGH PAIN** today.

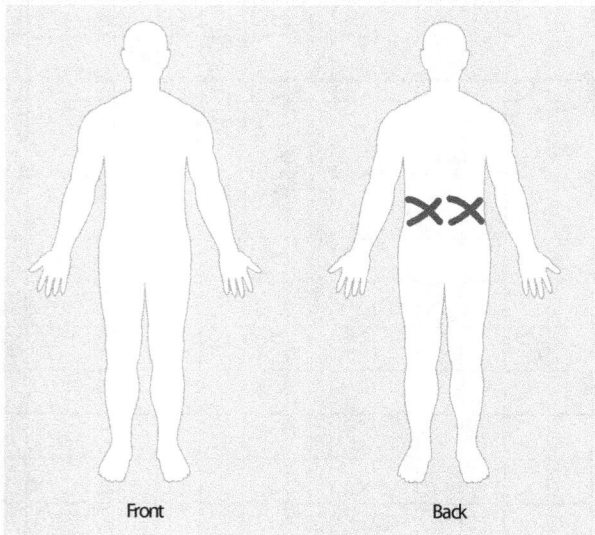

Front   Back

NON-DRUG THERAPIES
(other than prescription or other medicines)
Heating Pad

ACTIVITIES/EXERCISE
Yoga, Weight Lifting

What was your average level of pain today?

0 1 2 3 4 ⑤ 6 7 8 9 10

Other than prescription medicine, did you do anything else today to relieve the pain? _____NO ✓YES:
(Note any that you used.)
✓ Non-prescription drugs (e.g., acetaminophen, ibuprofen)
_____ Herbal remedies
✓ Hot or cold packs
✓ Exercise
✓ Changing position (such as lying down or elevating your legs)
_____ Physical therapy
_____ Massage
_____ Acupuncture
✓ Rest
_____ Prayer, meditation, guided imagery
_____ Relaxation technique (hypnosis, biofeedback)
_____ Creative technique (art or music therapy)
✓ Other (e.g., specific chiropractic manipulation, osteopathic treatments):
_____

Check any of these common side effects that you've noticed after taking your pain medicine:
_____ Drowsiness, sleepiness
_____ Nausea, vomiting, upset stomach
✓ Constipation
_____ Lack of appetite
✓ Other (describe):
Hallucinations

Did you sleep through the night? ✓NO_____YES

If not, how many times was your sleep disrupted? _2_

How many hours did you sleep during the night? _6 hrs_

COMMENTS AND MORE INFORMATION: Make notes for and about visits with your healthcare provider, side effects from treatments you may be experiencing, any problems you are having coping with your pain, and more about some of your previous answers or questions.

Pain medicine is helping, but I keep seeing shadows move in my peripheral vision.

Is there another medicine that works as well, but without hallucinations?

6 DAILY BODY PAIN DIAGRAM

Mark each place on the diagram where you have had pain today by placing an 'X', circling the location, or shading the area .

Describe the type of pain:

Shooting	Deep
Tingling	Sharp
Numbness	Burning / Hot
Cold	Aching
Surface Pain	Gnawing / Biting
Stabbing	Electrical / Shocks
Dull	Other_____
Stinging	

COMMENTS AND MORE INFORMATION:

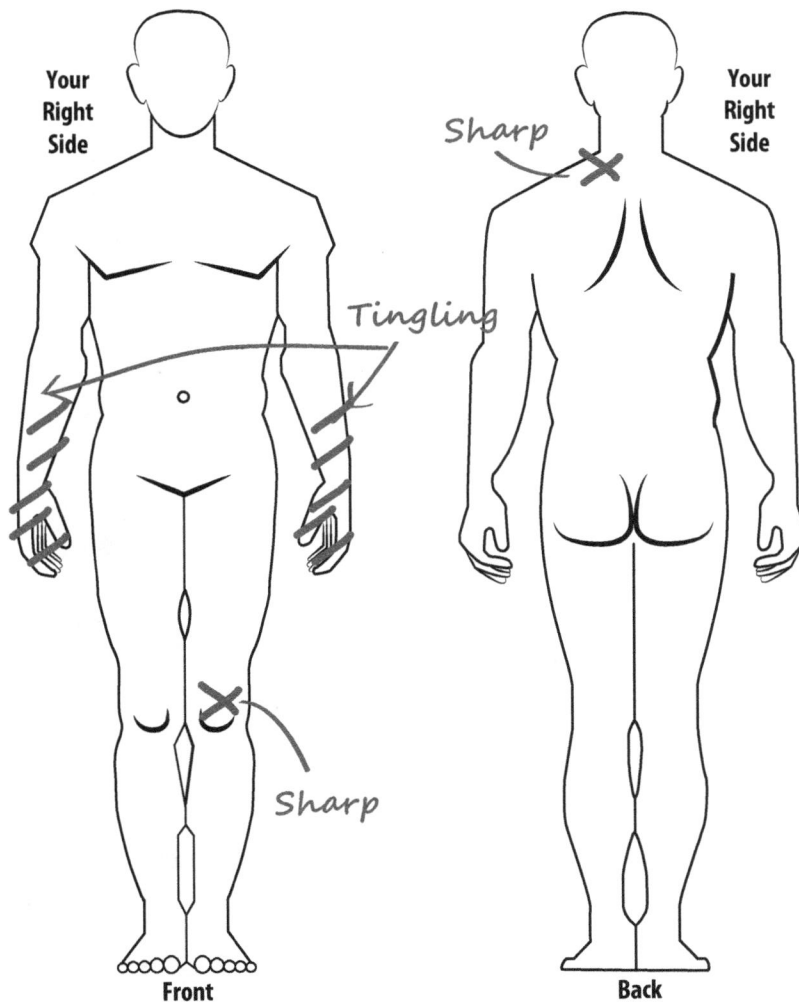

Your Right Side (front)

Tingling

Sharp

Front

Your Right Side (back)

Sharp

Back

DAILY SUMMARY EXAMPLES

MEDICAL HISTORY

1 PERSONAL
MEDICAL TEAM SUMMARY

NAME	PHONE	FAX	NOTES
ADDRESS			

NAME	PHONE	FAX	NOTES
ADDRESS			

NAME	PHONE	FAX	NOTES
ADDRESS			

NAME	PHONE	FAX	NOTES
ADDRESS			

NAME	PHONE	FAX	NOTES
ADDRESS			

1 PERSONAL
MEDICAL TEAM SUMMARY (CONTINUED)

NAME	PHONE	FAX	NOTES
ADDRESS			

NAME	PHONE	FAX	NOTES
ADDRESS			

NAME	PHONE	FAX	NOTES
ADDRESS			

NAME	PHONE	FAX	NOTES
ADDRESS			

NAME	PHONE	FAX	NOTES
ADDRESS			

2 CURRENT PERSCRIPTION MEDICATIONS

DRUG NAME	DOSAGE	FREQUENCY	TREATMENT FOR	SIDE EFFECTS

3 CURRENT OVER THE COUNTER MEDICATIONS (ASPIRIN, ETC.)

DRUG NAME	DOSAGE	FREQUENCY	TREATMENT FOR	SIDE EFFECTS

4 DRUG ALLERGY SUMMARY

DRUG NAME (include prescription and other medicines)	REACTION

5 PAIN SURVEY

Place a check (✓) in the appropriate box. ACTIVITY	None	Mild	Moderate	Severe	Unable	HELPFUL TREATMENTS / COMMENTS
Pain when performing the following?						
Bending						
Caring for Infirm Family						
Carrying Groceries						
Changing Position (Sit to Stand)						
Climbing Stairs						
Driving						
Extended Computer Use						
Feeding (Self)						
Household Chores						
Kneeling						
Lifting Children						
Lifting objects						
Pet Care						
Reading (Concentration)						
Self care - Bathing						
Self care - Dressing						
Self care - Shaving						
Sexual Activities						
Sleeping						
Sitting (Prolonged)						
Standing (Prolonged)						
Walking						
Yard Work						
Sports / Recreational Activities / Exercise						
List:						
List:						
List:						
List:						
List:						
List any other activities that cause pain:						

6 PERSONAL & FAMILY
HEALTH HISTORY (PAGE 1 OF 3)

Place a check (✓) in the corresponding box for each condition as it applies to you and you relatives.

CONDITION	YOU	YOUR MOTHER	YOUR FATHER	BROTHER(S)	SISTER(S)	MATERNAL GRANDMOTHER	MATERNAL GRANDFATHER	MATERNAL AUNT(S)/UNCLE(S)	PATERNAL GRANDMOTHER	PATERNAL GRANDFATHER	PATERNAL AUNT(S)/UNCLE(S)	COMMENTS
Head (Ear, Nose, Throat / Eyes / Jaw):												
Migraine Headaches												
Severe / Frequent Headaches												
Jaw Pain / TMJ												
Dizziness or Faintness												
Epilepsy / Seizures or Convulsions												
Near or Farsighted (Glasses)												
Glaucoma												
Cataracts												
Blindness												
Recurrent Ear Infecitons												
Deafness / Reduced Hearing												
Hay Fever												
Recurrent Sinusitis												
Overactive Thyroid (Hyperthyroidism)												
Underactive Thyroid (Hypothyroidism)												
Goiter												
Other:_____												
Psychological:												
Smoking												
Alcoholism												
Chemical Dependency												
Anxiety												
Serious Depression												
Post Traumatic Stress Disorder (PTSD)												
Nervous Breakdown												
Suicide / Attempt												
Bipolar Disorder												
Personality Disorder:_____												
Neurological (Nerves):												
Insomnia												
Sleep Apnea												
Peripheral Neuropathy												
Paralysis												
Orthopedic (Bones, Muscles, etc.):												
Arthritis / Swollen Joints / Rheumatism												
Osteoporosis												
Varicose Veins												
Connective Tissue Disorder												
Gout												
Broken Bones												
Cortisone Treatments												
Artificial Joints												
Swollen Feet or Ankles												
Back Problems / Injury												

6 HEALTH HISTORY (CONTINUED - PAGE 2 OF 3)

Place a check (✓) in the corresponding box for each condition as it applies to you and you relatives.

CONDITION	YOU	YOUR MOTHER	YOUR FATHER	BROTHER(S)	SISTER(S)	MATERNAL			PATERNAL			COMMENTS
						GRANDMOTHER	GRANDFATHER	AUNT(S) / UNCLE(S)	GRANDMOTHER	GRANDFATHER	AUNT(S) / UNCLE(S)	
Digestive (Stomache, Intestines, etc.):												
Hiatal Hernia / Chronic Heartburn												
Stomach or Duodenal Ulcer												
Hepatitis												
Cirrhosis / Liver Disease												
Gall Stones												
Irritable Bowel Syndrome (IBS)												
Ulcerative Colitis												
Diverticulitis (-osis)												
Polyps (Colon)												
Dysentery or Serious Diarrhea												
Rectal Trouble												
Hemorrhoids												
Recurrent Urinary Tract Infections (UTI)												
Frequent, Painful, or Difficult Urination												
Incontinence												
Kidney Stones												
Other Kidney Disease:_____												
Cardiopulmonary (Heart, Lungs, Blood):												
Phlebitis or Blood Clots / Emboli												
Anemia												
Asthma, Bronchitis or Emphysema												
Angina												
Heart Attack / Surgery												
Heart Murmur												
Enlarged Heart												
Coronary Heart Disease												
Artificial Heart Valves												
Pacemaker												
High Blood Pressure												
Low Blood Pressure												
Stroke / TIA												
Shortness of Breath / Chest Pain												
Asthma												
Chronic Bronchitis												
Cough, persistent or bloody												
Emphysema												
Tuberculosis												
Systemic Disease / Disorders:												
Diabetes												
Psoriasis, Eczema, or Rosacea												
Gonorrhea, Syphilis or Venereal Disease												
AIDS / HIV Infection												
Hepatitis Type _____												
Herpes Infection												

6 HEALTH HISTORY (CONTINUED - PAGE 3 OF 3)

Place a check (✓) in the corresponding box for each condition as it applies to you and you relatives.

Condition	You	Your Mother	Your Father	Brother(s)	Sister(s)	MATERNAL Grandmother	Grandfather	Aunt(s) / Uncle(s)	PATERNAL Grandmother	Grandfather	Aunt(s) / Uncle(s)	Comments
Systemic Disease / Disorders:												
Chicken Pox												
Shingles												
Mumps or Measles												
Rheumatic or Scarlet Fever												
Cancer (Type:_____)												
Cancer (Type:_____)												
Cancer (Type:_____)												
Women:												
Severe Menstrual Cramping												
Pre Menstrual Dimorphic Disorder (PMDD)												
Abnormal PAP												
Ovarian Cyst(s)												
Fibroids(s)												
Endometriosis / Adhesions												
Breast Lump(s)												
Men:												
Enlarged Prostate												
Erectile Dysfunction												
Other Medical Condition:												
Other:												
Other:												
Other:												
Other:												

7 MEDICATION SIDE EFFECTS

As you and your medical team develop new treatment plans, it will be especially helpful to record any side effects you experience as you add new treatments. This can help determine which types of treatments will work best for you.

Contact your care provider with any side effects.

MEDICATION NAME	DATE STARTED	DATE STOPPED	SIDE EFFECTS / COMMENTS

MONTHLY SUMMARIES

1 MONTHLY
PAIN OVERVIEW CHART

MONTH AT A GLANCE: Using the information documented on the daily pain graphing sheets, document the highest level of pain you experienced for each day. This will provide a means for recognizing patterns over a longer period of time.

YEAR _____

MONTH	1	2	3	4	5	6	7	8	9	10	11	12	13	14	15	16	17	18	19	20	21	22	23	24	25	26	27	28	29	30	31	Number of Days with Pain	Drug Change (✓)
JAN																																	
FEB																																	
MAR																																	
APR																																	
MAY																																	
JUNE																																	
JULY																																	
AUG																																	
SEPT																																	
OCT																																	
NOV																																	
DEC																																	

TYPE OF PAIN

WORST IMAGINABLE ■

SEVERE Ⓢ

MODERATE Ⓜ

TOLERABLE ⊠

COMMENTS AND MORE INFORMATION: Make notes for and about visits with your healthcare provider, side effects from treatments you may be experiencing, any problems you are having, and more about some of your previous answers or questions.

_____

_____

_____

_____

_____

_____

2 EXERCISE RECORD CHART

MONTH AT A GLANCE: Document the type of exercise you practiced for each day. This will provide a means for recognizing patterns over a long period of time.

YEAR																																Number of Days Exercised	Weight at End of the Month
MONTH	1	2	3	4	5	6	7	8	9	10	11	12	13	14	15	16	17	18	19	20	21	22	23	24	25	26	27	28	29	30	31		
JAN																																	
FEB																																	
MAR																																	
APR																																	
MAY																																	
JUNE																																	
JULY																																	
AUG																																	
SEPT																																	
OCT																																	
NOV																																	
DEC																																	

TYPE OF EXERCISE

Cardio ⊠

Weights ⊠

Cardio and Weights ▨

Other ⊘

COMMENTS AND MORE INFORMATION: Make notes for and about visits with your healthcare provider, side effects from treatments you may be experiencing, any problems you are having, and more about some of your previous answers or questions.

_____

_____

_____

_____

_____

_____

DAILY SUMMARIES

1 DAILY
TREATMENT PLAN

As you and your medical team develop new treatment plans, record your plan for the day including:
1.) New medications,
2.) Increases or decreases to medications,
3.) Exercises, physical therapy, or any other treatments,
4.) It will be especially helpful to record any side effects you experience as you add new treatments.
     This can help determine which types of treatments will work best for you.

Contact your care provider with any bad reactions or side effects to determine if you should discontinue the medication or treatment.

MEDICATION / TREATMENT	AMOUNT / TIME / COMMENTS

DAY_____ DATE_____ WEIGHT_____

INSTRUCTIONS:
1.) **Place an 'X'** on the chart below where the lines for the time of day and your level of pain meet.
2.) **Connect the points** on your DAILY PAIN CHART so your medical team can see when your status changed.
3.) **Refer to the EXAMPLES** in the front of this book for further direction.

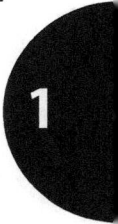

2 DAILY PAIN CHART

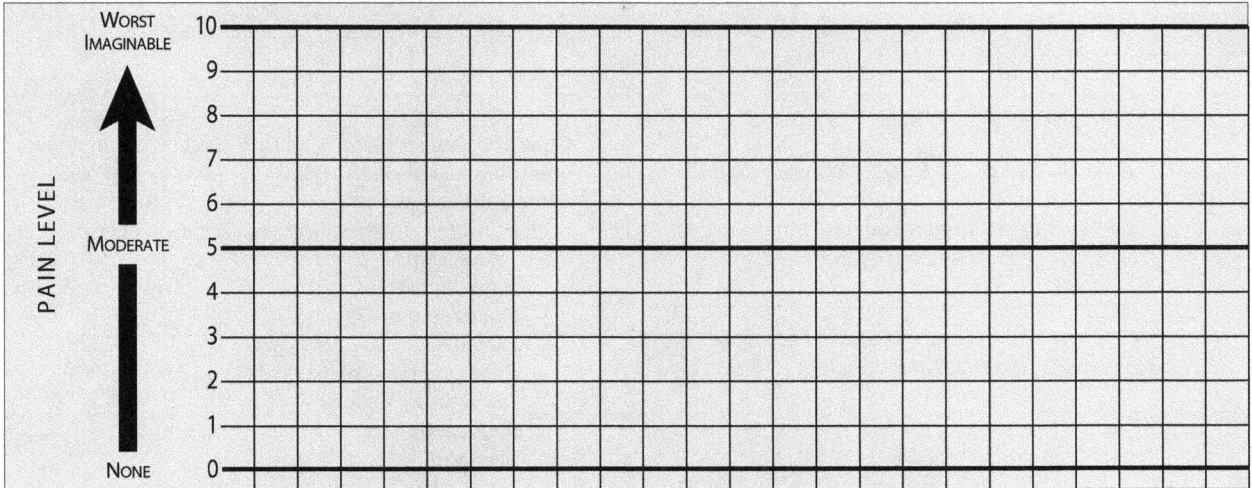

PAIN LEVEL

- WORST IMAGINABLE — 10
- 9
- 8
- 7
- 6
- MODERATE — 5
- 4
- 3
- 2
- 1
- NONE — 0

3 DAILY MEDICATION

MEDICINE NAME / DOSE — 6am, 7, 8, 9, 10, 11, 12pm, 1, 2, 3, 4, 5, 6pm, 7, 8, 9, 10, 11, 12am, 1, 2, 3, 4, 5

1
2
3
4
5
6
7
8
9

4 DAILY PHYSIOLOGY

6am, 7, 8, 9, 10, 11, 12pm, 1, 2, 3, 4, 5, 6pm, 7, 8, 9, 10, 11, 12am, 1, 2, 3, 4, 5

SLEEP
RESTROOM
NAUSEA / DIZZINESS
MEAL / SNACK
EXERCISE / PHYSICAL THERAPY
STRESS / ANXIETY
BLOOD PRESSURE
PULSE

5 DAILY
PAIN SUMMARY

Were there times during the day that you experienced unrelieved breakthrough pain? ____NO ____YES

How many times did this happen today?

   1 2 3 4 5 6 7 8 9 10 more than 10

Did any specific activity start your breakthrough pain?
____NO ____YES: What activities?

_____

Put an "X" on the body diagram to show each place you've had **BREAKTHROUGH PAIN** today.

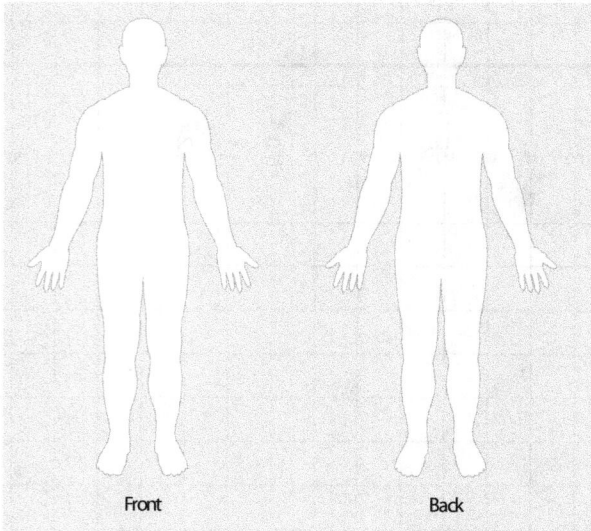

Front   Back

NON-DRUG THERAPIES
(other than prescription or other medicines)

_____

_____

ACTIVITIES/EXERCISE

_____

What was your average level of pain today?

  0 1 2 3 4 5 6 7 8 9 10

Other than prescription medicine, did you do anything else today to relieve the pain? ____NO ____YES:
(Note any that you used.)
____ Non-prescription drugs (e.g., acetaminophen, ibuprofen)
____ Herbal remedies
____ Hot or cold packs
____ Exercise
____ Changing position (such as lying down or elevating your legs)
____ Physical therapy
____ Massage
____ Acupuncture
____ Rest
____ Prayer, meditation, guided imagery
____ Relaxation technique (hypnosis, biofeedback)
____ Creative technique (art or music therapy)
____ Other (e.g., specific chiropractic manipulation, osteopathic treatments):

_____

Check any of these common side effects that you've noticed after taking your pain medicine:
____ Drowsiness, sleepiness
____ Nausea, vomiting, upset stomach
____ Constipation
____ Lack of appetite
____ Other (describe):

_____

Did you sleep through the night? ____NO____YES

If not, how many times was your sleep disrupted? _____

How many hours did you sleep during the night? _____

COMMENTS AND MORE INFORMATION: Make notes for and about visits with your healthcare provider, side effects from treatments you may be experiencing, any problems you are having coping with your pain, and more about some of your previous answers or questions.

_____

_____

_____

6 DAILY BODY PAIN DIAGRAM

Mark each place on the diagram where you have had pain today by placing an 'X', circling the location, or shading the area .

Describe the type of pain:

Shooting	Deep
Tingling	Sharp
Numbness	Burning / Hot
Cold	Aching
Surface Pain	Gnawing / Biting
Stabbing	Electrical / Shocks
Dull	Other_____
Stinging	

COMMENTS AND MORE INFORMATION:

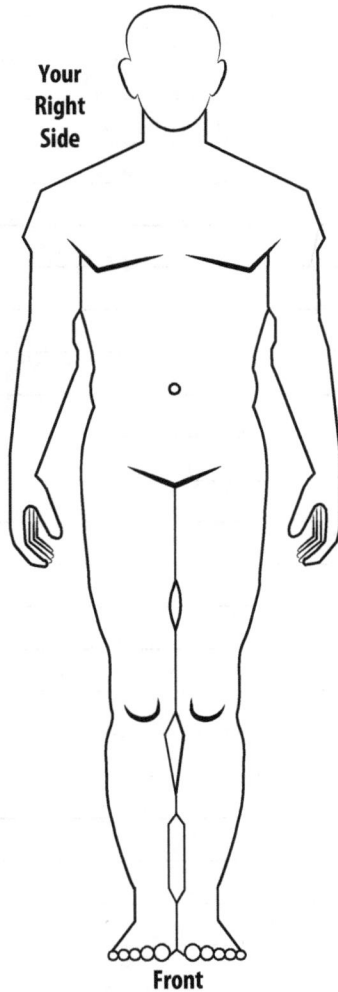

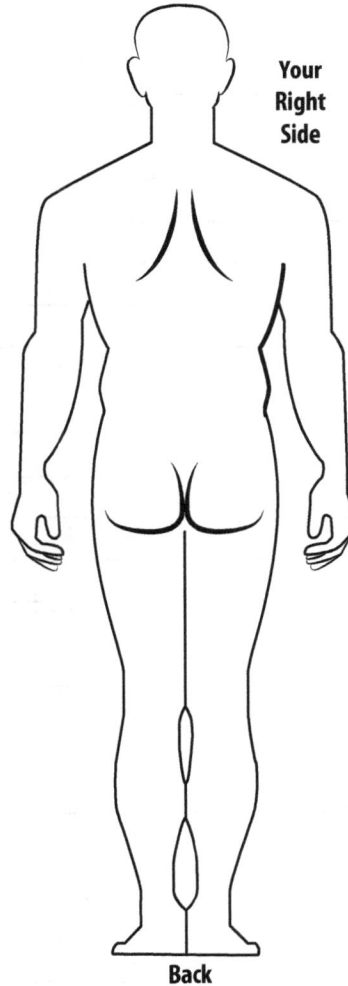

Your Right Side

Front

Your Right Side

Back

1 DAILY
TREATMENT PLAN

2

As you and your medical team develop new treatment plans, record your plan for the day including:
1.) New medications,
2.) Increases or decreases to medications,
3.) Exercises, physical therapy, or any other treatments,
4.) It will be especially helpful to record any side effects you experience as you add new treatments.
   This can help determine which types of treatments will work best for you.

Contact your care provider with any bad reactions or side effects to determine if you should discontinue the medication or treatment.

MEDICATION / TREATMENT	AMOUNT / TIME / COMMENTS

DAY_____ DATE_____ WEIGHT_____

INSTRUCTIONS:
1.) **Place an 'X'** on the chart below where the lines for the time of day and your level of pain meet.
2.) **Connect the points** on your DAILY PAIN CHART so your medical team can see when your status changed.
3.) **Refer to the EXAMPLES** in the front of this book for further direction.

2 DAILY PAIN CHART

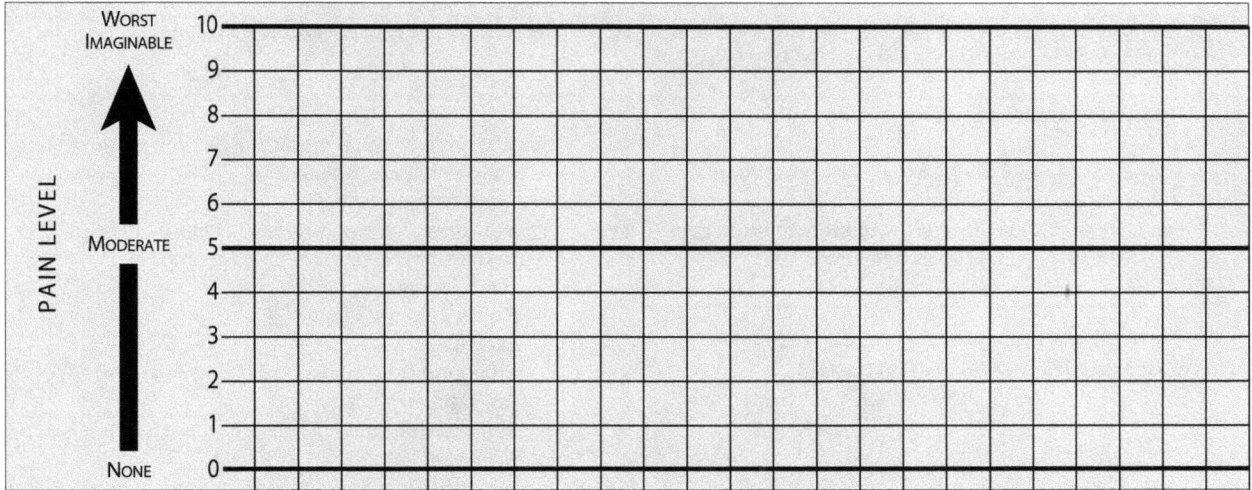

PAIN LEVEL

WORST IMAGINABLE	10
	9
	8
	7
	6
MODERATE	5
	4
	3
	2
	1
NONE	0

3 DAILY MEDICATION

MEDICINE NAME / DOSE

Time columns: 6am, 7, 8, 9, 10, 11, 12pm, 1, 2, 3, 4, 5, 6pm, 7, 8, 9, 10, 11, 12am, 1, 2, 3, 4, 5

1
2
3
4
5
6
7
8
9

4 DAILY PHYSIOLOGY

Time columns: 6am, 7, 8, 9, 10, 11, 12pm, 1, 2, 3, 4, 5, 6pm, 7, 8, 9, 10, 11, 12am, 1, 2, 3, 4, 5

SLEEP
RESTROOM
NAUSEA / DIZZINESS
MEAL / SNACK
EXERCISE / PHYSICAL THERAPY
STRESS / ANXIETY
BLOOD PRESSURE
PULSE

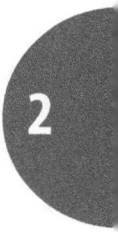

2

5 DAILY
PAIN SUMMARY

2

Were there times during the day that you experienced unrelieved breakthrough pain? ____NO ____YES

How many times did this happen today?

1 2 3 4 5 6 7 8 9 10 more than 10

Did any specific activity start your breakthrough pain? ____NO ____YES: What activities?

_____

Put an "X" on the body diagram to show each place you've had **BREAKTHROUGH PAIN** today.

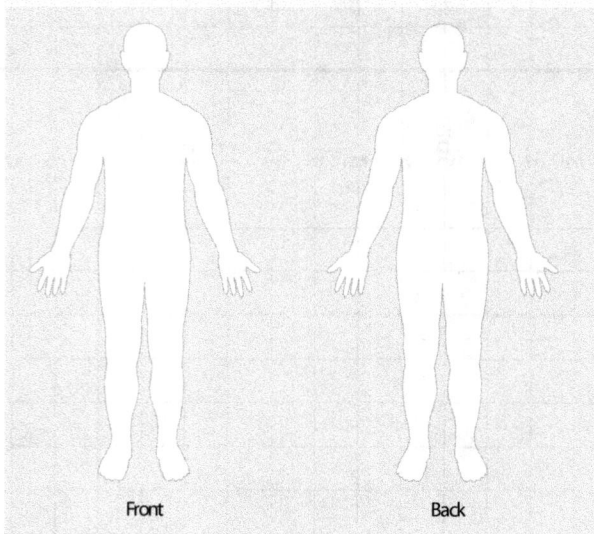

Front   Back

NON-DRUG THERAPIES
(other than prescription or other medicines)

_____

_____

ACTIVITIES/EXERCISE

_____

_____

What was your average level of pain today?

0 1 2 3 4 5 6 7 8 9 10

Other than prescription medicine, did you do anything else today to relieve the pain? ____NO ____YES:
(Note any that you used.)
____ Non-prescription drugs (e.g., acetaminophen, ibuprofen)
____ Herbal remedies
____ Hot or cold packs
____ Exercise
____ Changing position (such as lying down or elevating your legs)
____ Physical therapy
____ Massage
____ Acupuncture
____ Rest
____ Prayer, meditation, guided imagery
____ Relaxation technique (hypnosis, biofeedback)
____ Creative technique (art or music therapy)
____ Other (e.g., specific chiropractic manipulation, osteopathic treatments):

_____

Check any of these common side effects that you've noticed after taking your pain medicine:
____ Drowsiness, sleepiness
____ Nausea, vomiting, upset stomach
____ Constipation
____ Lack of appetite
____ Other (describe):

_____

Did you sleep through the night? ____NO____YES

If not, how many times was your sleep disrupted? _____

How many hours did you sleep during the night? _____

COMMENTS AND MORE INFORMATION: Make notes for and about visits with your healthcare provider, side effects from treatments you may be experiencing, any problems you are having coping with your pain, and more about some of your previous answers or questions.

_____

_____

_____

6 DAILY BODY PAIN DIAGRAM

Mark each place on the diagram where you have had pain today by placing an 'X', circling the location, or shading the area .

Describe the type of pain:

Shooting	Deep
Tingling	Sharp
Numbness	Burning / Hot
Cold	Aching
Surface Pain	Gnawing / Biting
Stabbing	Electrical / Shocks
Dull	Other_____
Stinging	

COMMENTS AND MORE INFORMATION:

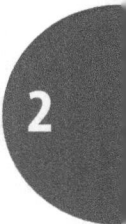

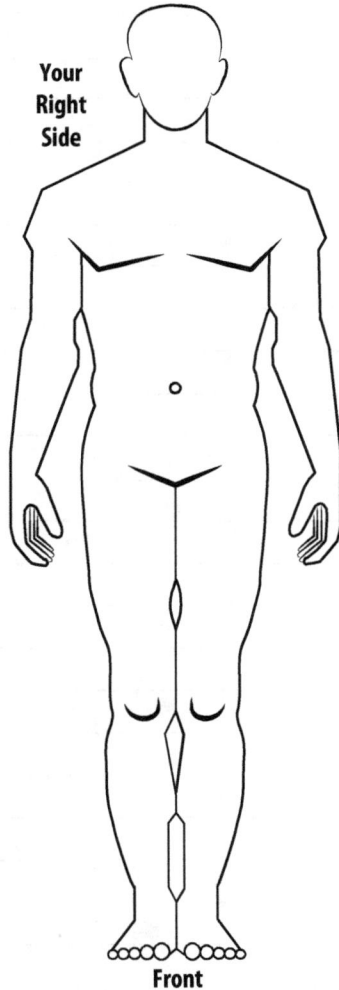

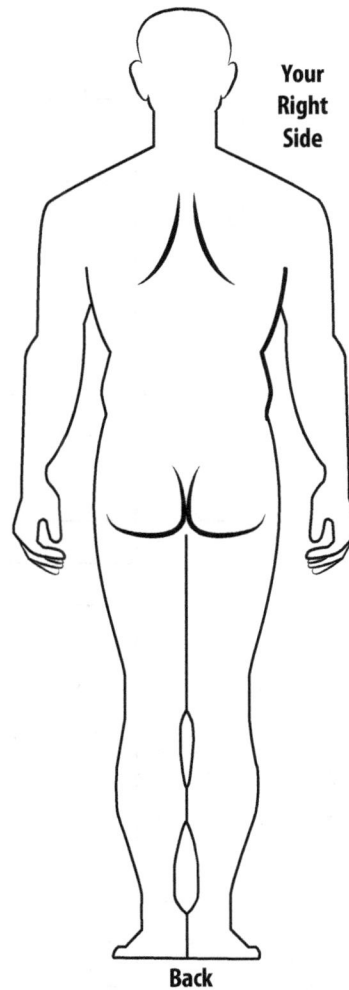

2

Your Right Side

Your Right Side

Front

Back

1 DAILY
TREATMENT PLAN

As you and your medical team develop new treatment plans, record your plan for the day including:
1.) New medications,
2.) Increases or decreases to medications,
3.) Exercises, physical therapy, or any other treatments,
4.) It will be especially helpful to record any side effects you experience as you add new treatments.
   This can help determine which types of treatments will work best for you.

Contact your care provider with any bad reactions or side effects to determine if you should discontinue the medication or treatment.

MEDICATION / TREATMENT	AMOUNT / TIME / COMMENTS

DAY_____ DATE_____ WEIGHT_____

INSTRUCTIONS:
1.) **Place an 'X'** on the chart below where the lines for the time of day and your level of pain meet.
2.) **Connect the points** on your DAILY PAIN CHART so your medical team can see when your status changed.
3.) **Refer to the EXAMPLES** in the front of this book for further direction.

2 DAILY PAIN CHART

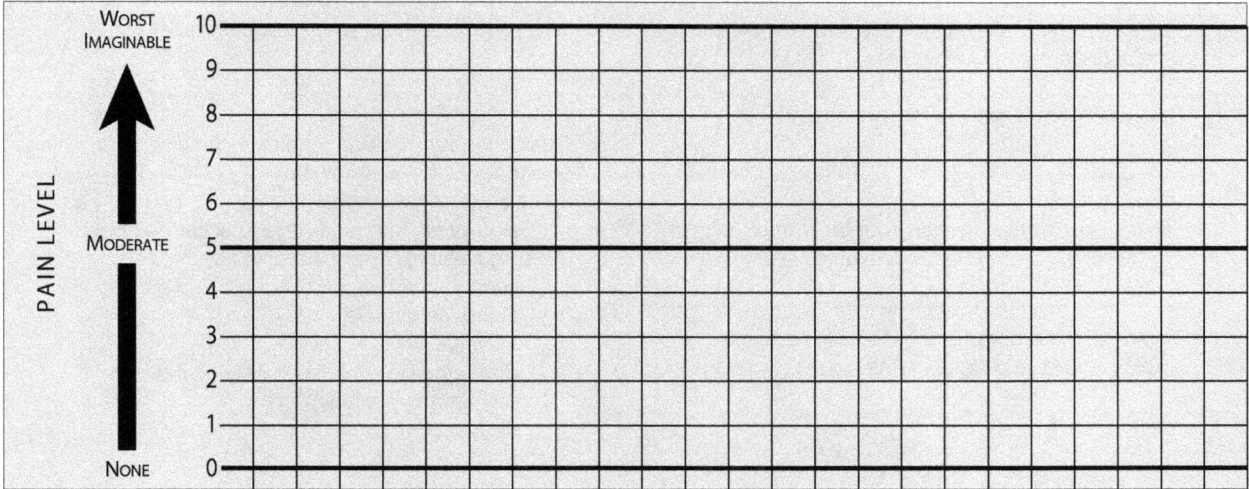

WORST IMAGINABLE — 10
9
8
7
6
MODERATE — 5
4
3
2
1
NONE — 0

PAIN LEVEL

3 DAILY MEDICATION

MEDICINE NAME / DOSE

6am 7 8 9 10 11 12pm 1 2 3 4 5 6pm 7 8 9 10 11 12am 1 2 3 4 5

1
2
3
4
5
6
7
8
9

4 DAILY PHYSIOLOGY

6am 7 8 9 10 11 12pm 1 2 3 4 5 6pm 7 8 9 10 11 12am 1 2 3 4 5

SLEEP
RESTROOM
NAUSEA / DIZZINESS
MEAL / SNACK
EXERCISE / PHYSICAL THERAPY
STRESS / ANXIETY
BLOOD PRESSURE
PULSE

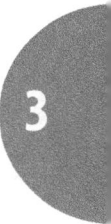

3

5 DAILY
PAIN SUMMARY

Were there times during the day that you experienced unrelieved breakthrough pain? ____NO ____YES

How many times did this happen today?

1 2 3 4 5 6 7 8 9 10 more than 10

Did any specific activity start your breakthrough pain?
____NO ____YES: What activities?

_____

Put an "X" on the body diagram to show each place you've had **BREAKTHROUGH PAIN** today.

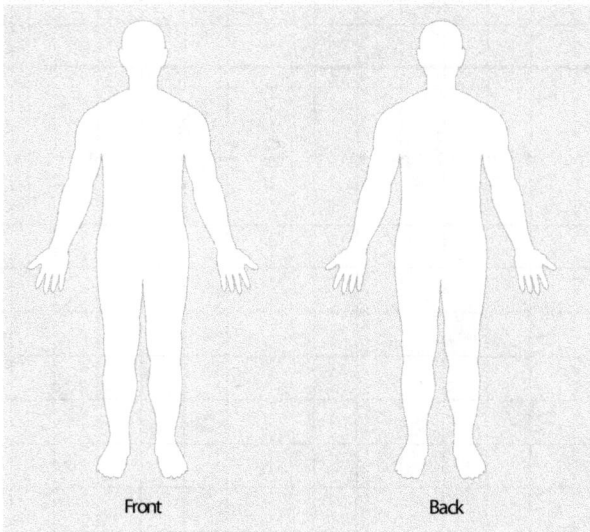

Front   Back

NON-DRUG THERAPIES
(other than prescription or other medicines)

_____

ACTIVITIES/EXERCISE

_____

What was your average level of pain today?

0 1 2 3 4 5 6 7 8 9 10

Other than prescription medicine, did you do anything else today to relieve the pain? ____NO ____YES:
(Note any that you used.)
____ Non-prescription drugs (e.g., acetaminophen, ibuprofen)
____ Herbal remedies
____ Hot or cold packs
____ Exercise
____ Changing position (such as lying down or elevating your legs)
____ Physical therapy
____ Massage
____ Acupuncture
____ Rest
____ Prayer, meditation, guided imagery
____ Relaxation technique (hypnosis, biofeedback)
____ Creative technique (art or music therapy)
____ Other (e.g., specific chiropractic manipulation, osteopathic treatments):

_____

Check any of these common side effects that you've noticed after taking your pain medicine:
____ Drowsiness, sleepiness
____ Nausea, vomiting, upset stomach
____ Constipation
____ Lack of appetite
____ Other (describe):

_____

Did you sleep through the night? ____NO____YES

If not, how many times was your sleep disrupted? _____

How many hours did you sleep during the night? _____

COMMENTS AND MORE INFORMATION: Make notes for and about visits with your healthcare provider, side effects from treatments you may be experiencing, any problems you are having coping with your pain, and more about some of your previous answers or questions.

_____

_____

_____

6 DAILY BODY PAIN DIAGRAM

Mark each place on the diagram where you have had pain today by placing an 'X', circling the location, or shading the area .

Describe the type of pain:

Shooting	Deep
Tingling	Sharp
Numbness	Burning / Hot
Cold	Aching
Surface Pain	Gnawing / Biting
Stabbing	Electrical / Shocks
Dull	Other_____
Stinging	

COMMENTS AND MORE INFORMATION:

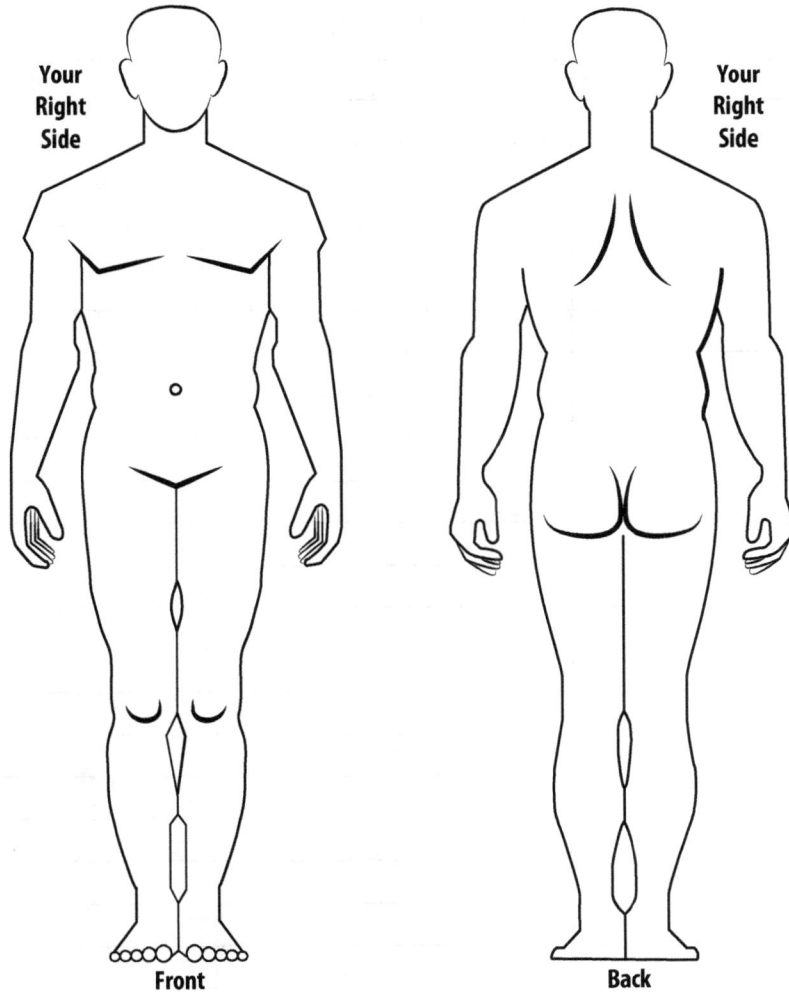

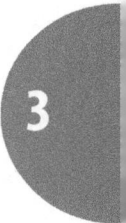

3

Your
Right
Side

Front

Your
Right
Side

Back

1 DAILY
TREATMENT PLAN

As you and your medical team develop new treatment plans, record your plan for the day including:
1.) New medications,
2.) Increases or decreases to medications,
3.) Exercises, physical therapy, or any other treatments,
4.) It will be especially helpful to record any side effects you experience as you add new treatments.
   This can help determine which types of treatments will work best for you.

Contact your care provider with any bad reactions or side effects to determine if you should discontinue the medication or treatment.

MEDICATION / TREATMENT	AMOUNT / TIME / COMMENTS

4

DAY_____ DATE_____ WEIGHT_____

INSTRUCTIONS:
1.) **Place an 'X'** on the chart below where the lines for the time of day and your level of pain meet.
2.) **Connect the points** on your DAILY PAIN CHART so your medical team can see when your status changed.
3.) **Refer to the EXAMPLES** in the front of this book for further direction.

2 DAILY PAIN CHART

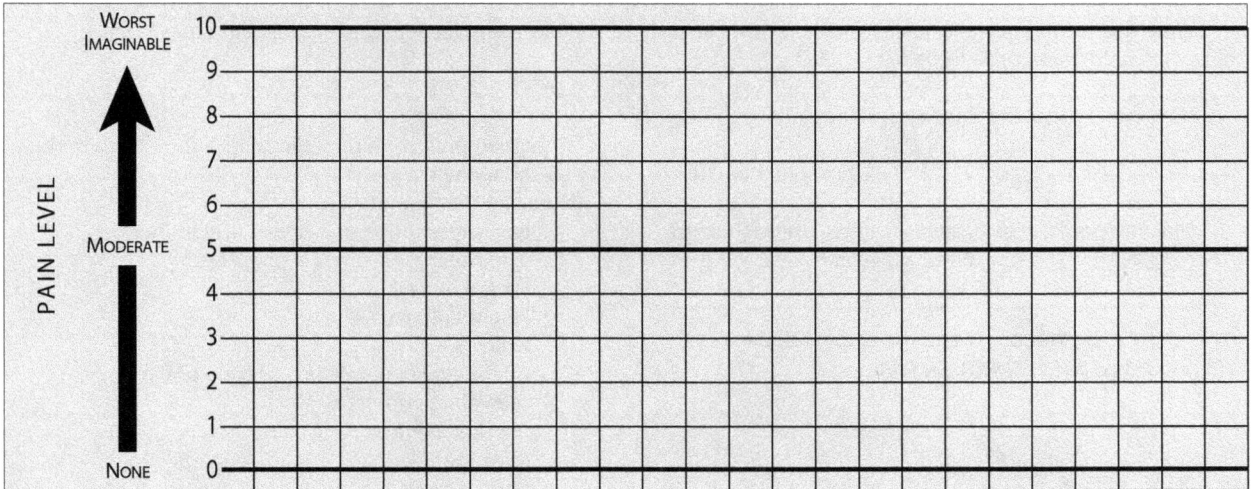

PAIN LEVEL

WORST IMAGINABLE	10
	9
	8
	7
	6
MODERATE	5
	4
	3
	2
	1
NONE	0

3 DAILY MEDICATION

MEDICINE NAME / DOSE

6am 7 8 9 10 11 12pm 1 2 3 4 5 6pm 7 8 9 10 11 12am 1 2 3 4 5

1
2
3
4
5
6
7
8
9

4

4 DAILY PHYSIOLOGY

6am 7 8 9 10 11 12pm 1 2 3 4 5 6pm 7 8 9 10 11 12am 1 2 3 4 5

SLEEP
RESTROOM
NAUSEA / DIZZINESS
MEAL / SNACK
EXERCISE / PHYSICAL THERAPY
STRESS / ANXIETY
BLOOD PRESSURE
PULSE

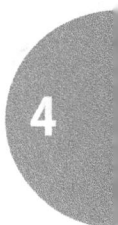

5 DAILY
PAIN SUMMARY

Were there times during the day that you experienced unrelieved breakthrough pain? ____NO ____YES

How many times did this happen today?

1 2 3 4 5 6 7 8 9 10 more than 10

Did any specific activity start your breakthrough pain?
____NO ____YES: What activities?

_____

Put an "X" on the body diagram to show each place you've had *BREAKTHROUGH PAIN* today.

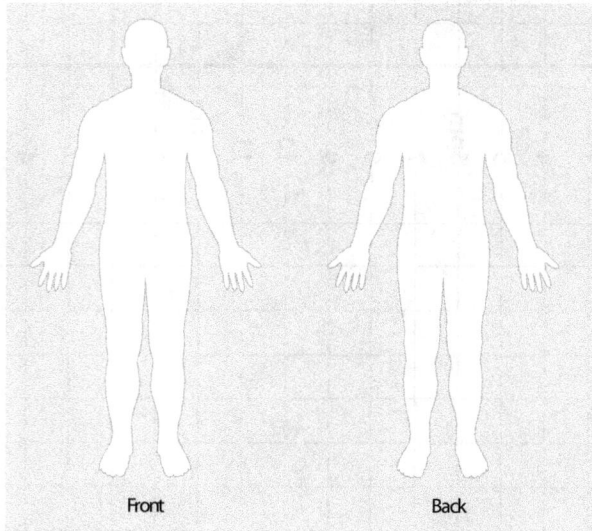

Front   Back

NON-DRUG THERAPIES
(other than prescription or other medicines)

_____

_____

ACTIVITIES/EXERCISE

_____

What was your average level of pain today?

0 1 2 3 4 5 6 7 8 9 10

Other than prescription medicine, did you do anything else today to relieve the pain? ____NO ____YES: (Note any that you used.)
____ Non-prescription drugs (e.g., acetaminophen, ibuprofen)
____ Herbal remedies
____ Hot or cold packs
____ Exercise
____ Changing position (such as lying down or elevating your legs)
____ Physical therapy
____ Massage
____ Acupuncture
____ Rest
____ Prayer, meditation, guided imagery
____ Relaxation technique (hypnosis, biofeedback)
____ Creative technique (art or music therapy)
____ Other (e.g., specific chiropractic manipulation, osteopathic treatments):

_____

Check any of these common side effects that you've noticed after taking your pain medicine:
____ Drowsiness, sleepiness
____ Nausea, vomiting, upset stomach
____ Constipation
____ Lack of appetite
____ Other (describe):

_____

Did you sleep through the night? ____NO____YES

If not, how many times was your sleep disrupted? _____

How many hours did you sleep during the night? _____

COMMENTS AND MORE INFORMATION: Make notes for and about visits with your healthcare provider, side effects from treatments you may be experiencing, any problems you are having coping with your pain, and more about some of your previous answers or questions.

_____

_____

_____

6 DAILY BODY PAIN DIAGRAM

Mark each place on the diagram where you have had pain today by placing an 'X', circling the location, or shading the area .

Describe the type of pain:

Shooting	Deep
Tingling	Sharp
Numbness	Burning / Hot
Cold	Aching
Surface Pain	Gnawing / Biting
Stabbing	Electrical / Shocks
Dull	Other_____
Stinging	

COMMENTS AND MORE INFORMATION:

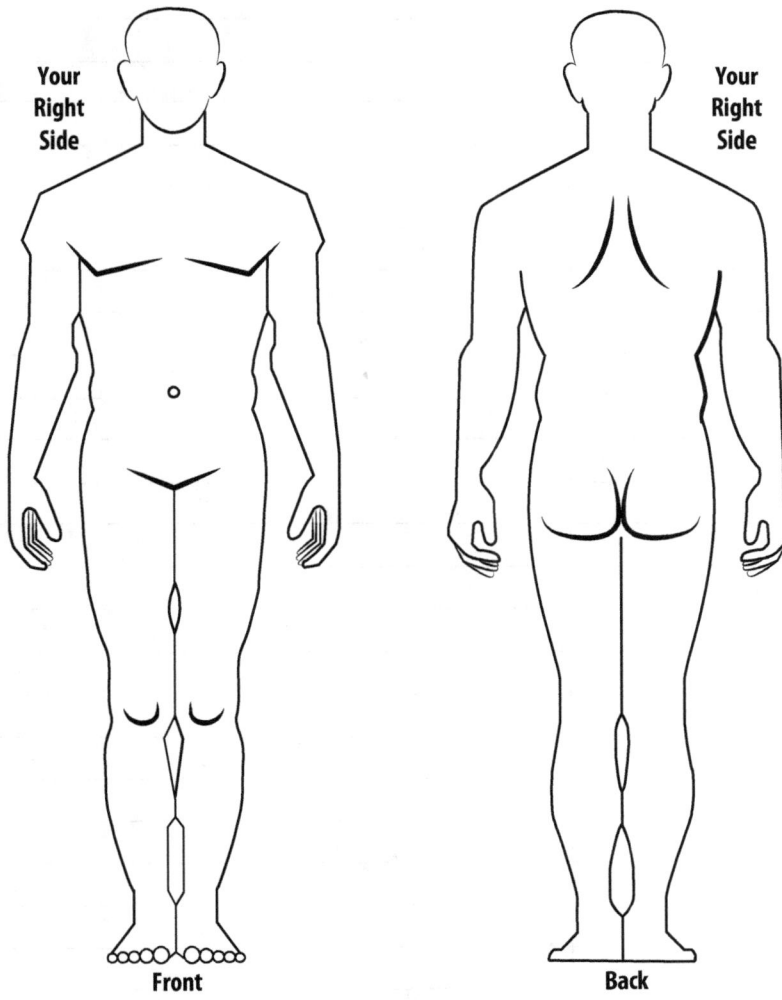

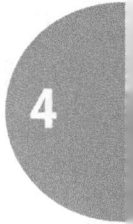

Your Right Side

Your Right Side

4

Front

Back

1 DAILY
TREATMENT PLAN

As you and your medical team develop new treatment plans, record your plan for the day including:
1.) New medications,
2.) Increases or decreases to medications,
3.) Exercises, physical therapy, or any other treatments,
4.) It will be especially helpful to record any side effects you experience as you add new treatments.
    This can help determine which types of treatments will work best for you.

Contact your care provider with any bad reactions or side effects to determine if you should discontinue the medication or treatment.

MEDICATION / TREATMENT	AMOUNT / TIME / COMMENTS

5

DAY_____ DATE_____ WEIGHT_____

INSTRUCTIONS:
1.) **Place an 'X'** on the chart below where the lines for the time of day and your level of pain meet.
2.) **Connect the points** on your DAILY PAIN CHART so your medical team can see when your status changed.
3.) **Refer to the EXAMPLES** in the front of this book for further direction.

2 DAILY PAIN CHART

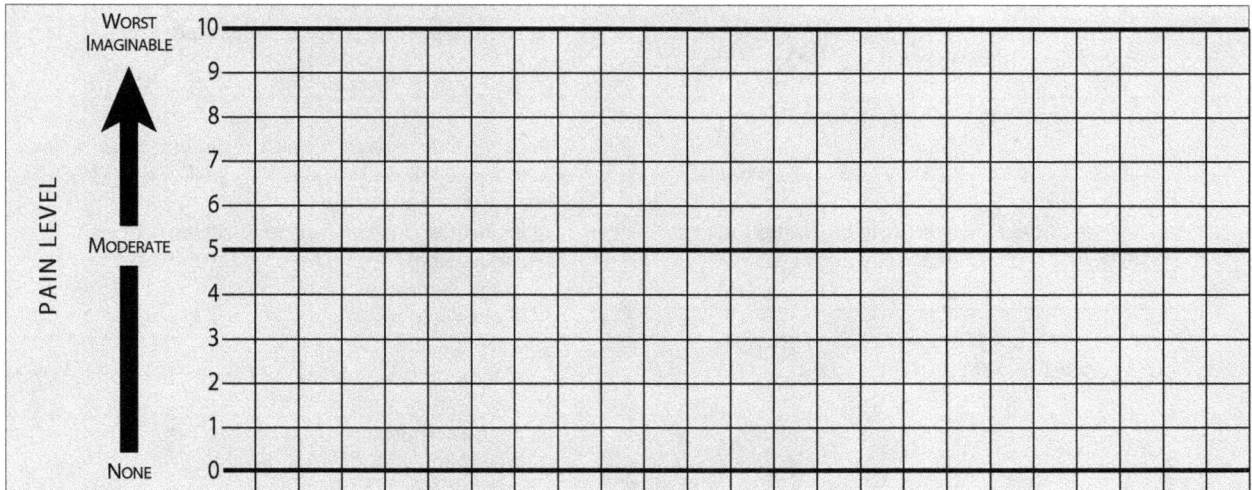

PAIN LEVEL

WORST IMAGINABLE	10
	9
	8
	7
	6
MODERATE	5
	4
	3
	2
	1
NONE	0

3 DAILY MEDICATION

MEDICINE NAME / DOSE

6am 7 8 9 10 11 12pm 1 2 3 4 5 6pm 7 8 9 10 11 12am 1 2 3 4 5

1
2
3
4
5
6
7
8
9

4 DAILY PHYSIOLOGY

6am 7 8 9 10 11 12pm 1 2 3 4 5 6pm 7 8 9 10 11 12am 1 2 3 4 5

SLEEP
RESTROOM
NAUSEA / DIZZINESS
MEAL / SNACK
EXERCISE / PHYSICAL THERAPY
STRESS / ANXIETY
BLOOD PRESSURE
PULSE

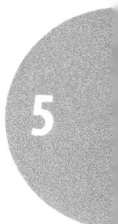

5

5 DAILY
PAIN SUMMARY

Were there times during the day that you experienced unrelieved breakthrough pain? ____NO ____YES

How many times did this happen today?

  1 2 3 4 5 6 7 8 9 10 more than 10

Did any specific activity start your breakthrough pain?
____NO ____YES: What activities?

_____

Put an "X" on the body diagram to show each place you've had **BREAKTHROUGH PAIN** today.

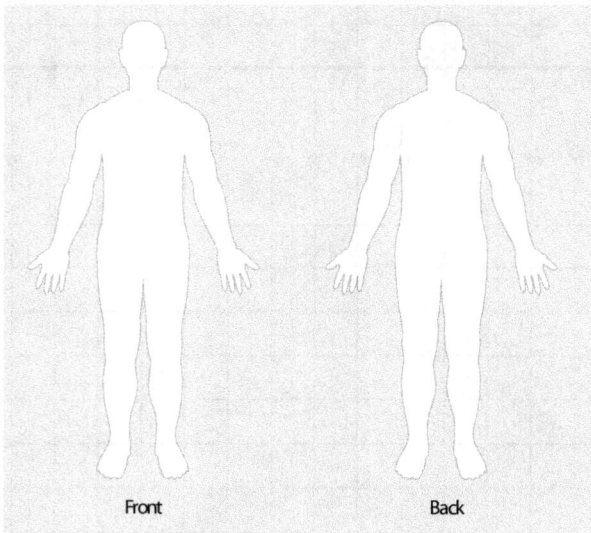

Front   Back

NON-DRUG THERAPIES
(other than prescription or other medicines)

_____

_____

ACTIVITIES/EXERCISE

_____

What was your average level of pain today?

  0 1 2 3 4 5 6 7 8 9 10

Other than prescription medicine, did you do anything else today to relieve the pain? ____NO ____YES:
(Note any that you used.)
____ Non-prescription drugs (e.g., acetaminophen, ibuprofen)
____ Herbal remedies
____ Hot or cold packs
____ Exercise
____ Changing position (such as lying down or elevating your legs)
____ Physical therapy
____ Massage
____ Acupuncture
____ Rest
____ Prayer, meditation, guided imagery
____ Relaxation technique (hypnosis, biofeedback)
____ Creative technique (art or music therapy)
____ Other (e.g., specific chiropractic manipulation, osteopathic treatments):

_____

Check any of these common side effects that you've noticed after taking your pain medicine:
____ Drowsiness, sleepiness
____ Nausea, vomiting, upset stomach
____ Constipation
____ Lack of appetite
____ Other (describe):

_____

Did you sleep through the night? ____NO____YES

If not, how many times was your sleep disrupted? _____

How many hours did you sleep during the night? _____

COMMENTS AND MORE INFORMATION: Make notes for and about visits with your healthcare provider, side effects from treatments you may be experiencing, any problems you are having coping with your pain, and more about some of your previous answers or questions.

_____

_____

_____

6 DAILY BODY PAIN DIAGRAM

Mark each place on the diagram where you have had pain today by placing an 'X', circling the location, or shading the area .

Describe the type of pain:

Shooting   Deep
Tingling   Sharp
Numbness   Burning / Hot
Cold   Aching
Surface Pain   Gnawing / Biting
Stabbing   Electrical / Shocks
Dull   Other_____
Stinging

COMMENTS AND MORE INFORMATION:

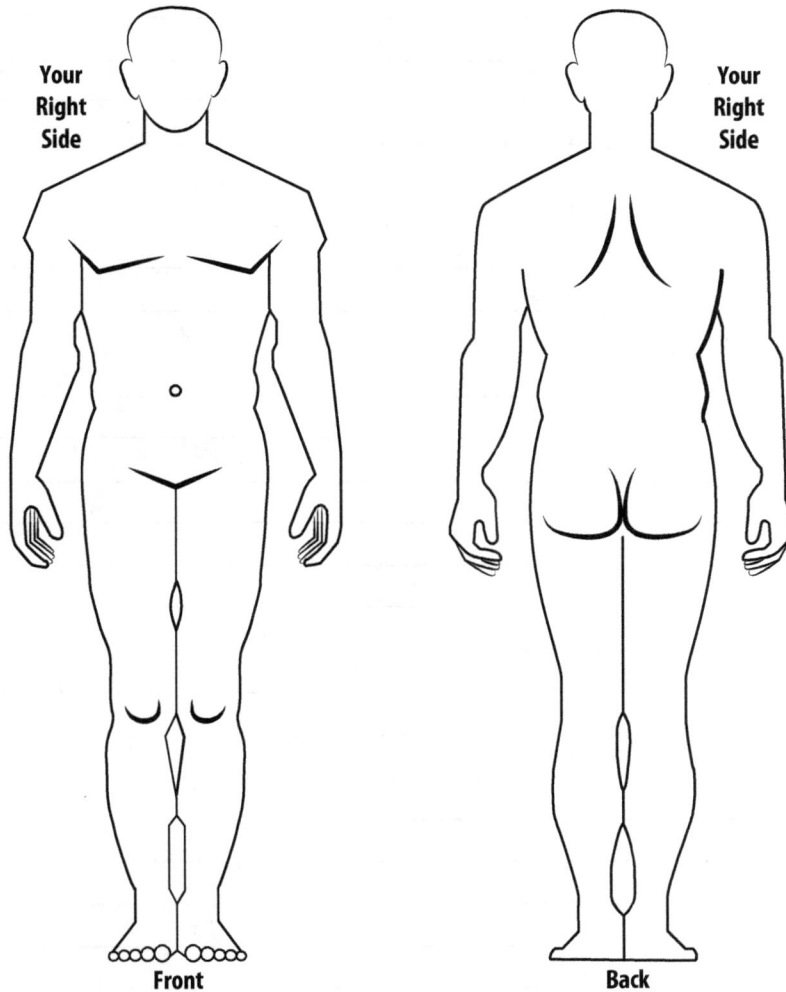

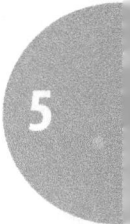

Your Right Side

Your Right Side

Front

Back

5

1 DAILY
TREATMENT PLAN

As you and your medical team develop new treatment plans, record your plan for the day including:

1.) New medications,
2.) Increases or decreases to medications,
3.) Exercises, physical therapy, or any other treatments,
4.) It will be especially helpful to record any side effects you experience as you add new treatments.
    This can help determine which types of treatments will work best for you.

Contact your care provider with any bad reactions or side effects to determine if you should discontinue the medication or treatment.

MEDICATION / TREATMENT	AMOUNT / TIME / COMMENTS

6

INSTRUCTIONS:
1.) **Place an 'X'** on the chart below where the lines for the time of day and your level of pain meet.
2.) **Connect the points** on your DAILY PAIN CHART so your medical team can see when your status changed.
3.) **Refer to the EXAMPLES** in the front of this book for further direction.

DAY_____ DATE_____ WEIGHT_____

2 DAILY PAIN CHART

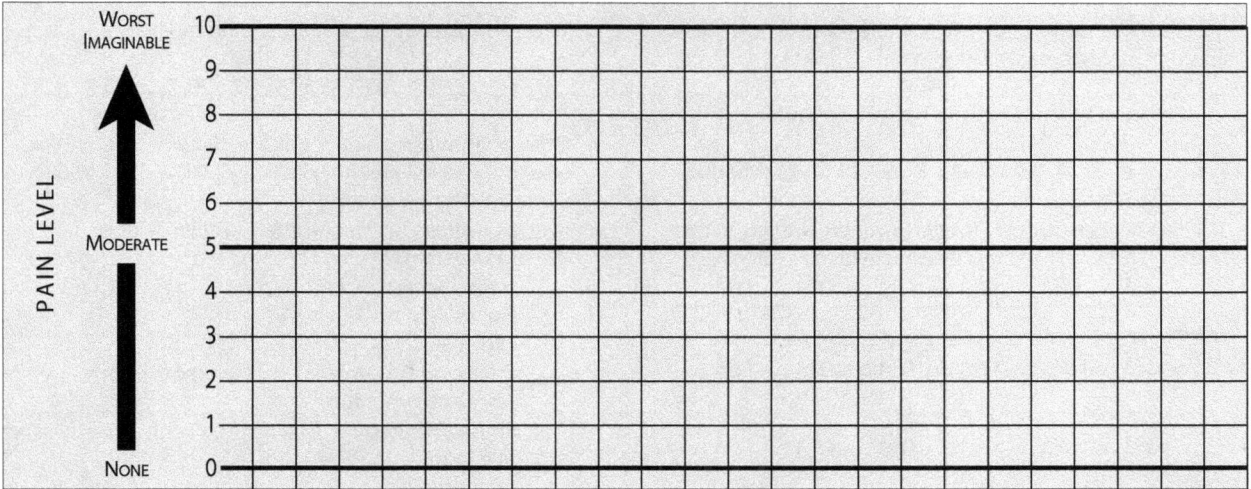

PAIN LEVEL

WORST IMAGINABLE	10
	9
	8
	7
	6
MODERATE	5
	4
	3
	2
	1
NONE	0

3 DAILY MEDICATION

MEDICINE NAME / DOSE

6am 7 8 9 10 11 12pm 1 2 3 4 5 6pm 7 8 9 10 11 12am 1 2 3 4 5

1
2
3
4
5
6
7
8
9

4 DAILY PHYSIOLOGY

6am 7 8 9 10 11 12pm 1 2 3 4 5 6pm 7 8 9 10 11 12am 1 2 3 4 5

SLEEP
RESTROOM
NAUSEA / DIZZINESS
MEAL / SNACK
EXERCISE / PHYSICAL THERAPY
STRESS / ANXIETY
BLOOD PRESSURE
PULSE

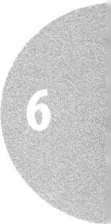

6

5 DAILY
PAIN SUMMARY

Were there times during the day that you experienced unrelieved breakthrough pain? ____NO ____YES

How many times did this happen today?

   1 2 3 4 5 6 7 8 9 10 more than 10

Did any specific activity start your breakthrough pain? ____NO ____YES: What activities?

_____

Put an "X" on the body diagram to show each place you've had **BREAKTHROUGH PAIN** today.

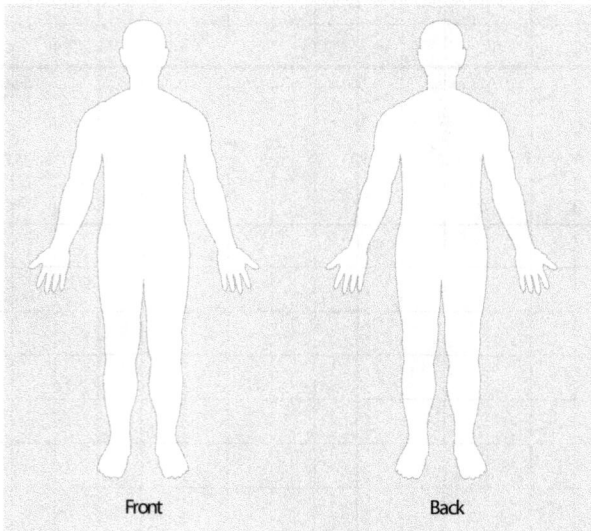

Front   Back

NON-DRUG THERAPIES
(other than prescription or other medicines)

_____

_____

ACTIVITIES/EXERCISE

_____

What was your average level of pain today?

  0 1 2 3 4 5 6 7 8 9 10

Other than prescription medicine, did you do anything else today to relieve the pain? ____NO ____YES: (Note any that you used.)
____ Non-prescription drugs (e.g., acetaminophen, ibuprofen)
____ Herbal remedies
____ Hot or cold packs
____ Exercise
____ Changing position (such as lying down or elevating your legs)
____ Physical therapy
____ Massage
____ Acupuncture
____ Rest
____ Prayer, meditation, guided imagery
____ Relaxation technique (hypnosis, biofeedback)
____ Creative technique (art or music therapy)
____ Other (e.g., specific chiropractic manipulation, osteopathic treatments):

_____

Check any of these common side effects that you've noticed after taking your pain medicine:
____ Drowsiness, sleepiness
____ Nausea, vomiting, upset stomach
____ Constipation
____ Lack of appetite
____ Other (describe):

_____

Did you sleep through the night? ____NO____YES

If not, how many times was your sleep disrupted? _____

How many hours did you sleep during the night? _____

COMMENTS AND MORE INFORMATION: Make notes for and about visits with your healthcare provider, side effects from treatments you may be experiencing, any problems you are having coping with your pain, and more about some of your previous answers or questions.

_____

_____

_____

6 DAILY BODY PAIN DIAGRAM

Mark each place on the diagram where you have had pain today by placing an 'X', circling the location, or shading the area .

Describe the type of pain:

Shooting   Deep
Tingling   Sharp
Numbness   Burning / Hot
Cold   Aching
Surface Pain   Gnawing / Biting
Stabbing   Electrical / Shocks
Dull   Other_____
Stinging

COMMENTS AND MORE INFORMATION:

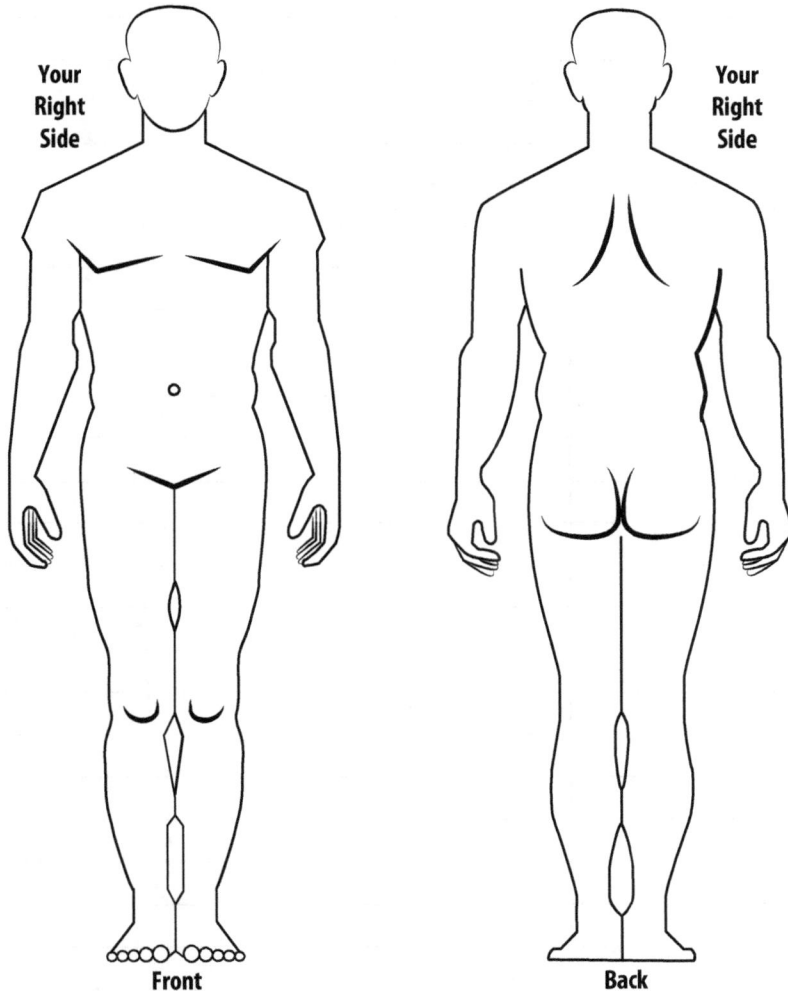

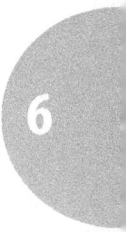

Your Right Side

Your Right Side

Front

Back

6

1 DAILY
TREATMENT PLAN

As you and your medical team develop new treatment plans, record your plan for the day including:
1.) New medications,
2.) Increases or decreases to medications,
3.) Exercises, physical therapy, or any other treatments,
4.) It will be especially helpful to record any side effects you experience as you add new treatments.
   This can help determine which types of treatments will work best for you.

Contact your care provider with any bad reactions or side effects to determine if you should discontinue the medication or treatment.

MEDICATION / TREATMENT	AMOUNT / TIME / COMMENTS

DAY_____ DATE_____ WEIGHT_____

INSTRUCTIONS:
1.) **Place an 'X'** on the chart below where the lines for the time of day and your level of pain meet.
2.) **Connect the points** on your DAILY PAIN CHART so your medical team can see when your status changed.
3.) **Refer to the EXAMPLES** in the front of this book for further direction.

2 DAILY PAIN CHART

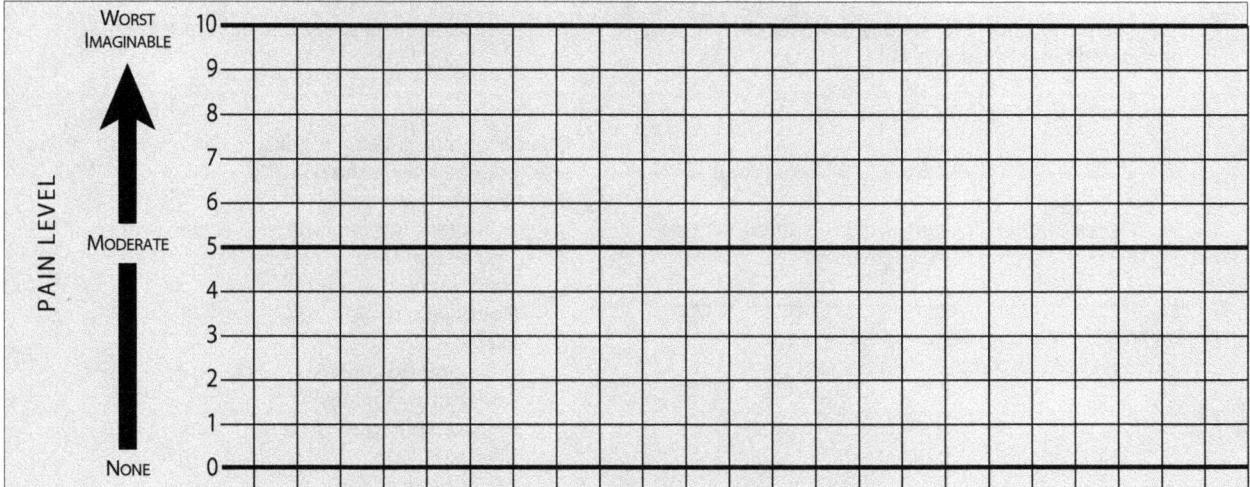

PAIN LEVEL

WORST IMAGINABLE — 10
9
8
7
6
MODERATE — 5
4
3
2
1
NONE — 0

3 DAILY MEDICATION

MEDICINE NAME / DOSE

	6am	7	8	9	10	11	12pm	1	2	3	4	5	6pm	7	8	9	10	11	12am	1	2	3	4	5
1																								
2																								
3																								
4																								
5																								
6																								
7																								
8																								
9																								

4 DAILY PHYSIOLOGY

	6am	7	8	9	10	11	12pm	1	2	3	4	5	6pm	7	8	9	10	11	12am	1	2	3	4	5
SLEEP																								
RESTROOM																								
NAUSEA / DIZZINESS																								
MEAL / SNACK																								
EXERCISE / PHYSICAL THERAPY																								
STRESS / ANXIETY																								
BLOOD PRESSURE																								
PULSE																								

7

5 DAILY
PAIN SUMMARY

Were there times during the day that you experienced unrelieved breakthrough pain? _____NO _____YES

How many times did this happen today?

1 2 3 4 5 6 7 8 9 10   more than 10

Did any specific activity start your breakthrough pain? _____NO _____YES: What activities?

_____

Put an "X" on the body diagram to show each place you've had **BREAKTHROUGH PAIN** today.

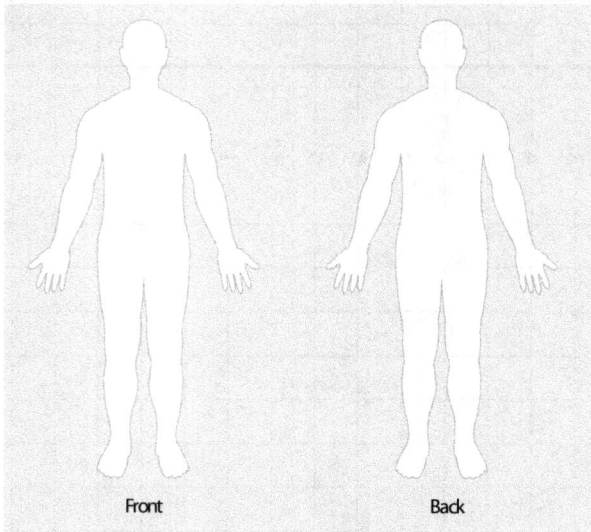

Front   Back

NON-DRUG THERAPIES
(other than prescription or other medicines)

_____

_____

ACTIVITIES/EXERCISE

_____

_____

What was your average level of pain today?

0 1 2 3 4 5 6 7 8 9 10

Other than prescription medicine, did you do anything else today to relieve the pain? _____NO _____YES: (Note any that you used.)
____ Non-prescription drugs (e.g., acetaminophen, ibuprofen)
____ Herbal remedies
____ Hot or cold packs
____ Exercise
____ Changing position (such as lying down or elevating your legs)
____ Physical therapy
____ Massage
____ Acupuncture
____ Rest
____ Prayer, meditation, guided imagery
____ Relaxation technique (hypnosis, biofeedback)
____ Creative technique (art or music therapy)
____ Other (e.g., specific chiropractic manipulation, osteopathic treatments):

_____

Check any of these common side effects that you've noticed after taking your pain medicine:
____ Drowsiness, sleepiness
____ Nausea, vomiting, upset stomach
____ Constipation
____ Lack of appetite
____ Other (describe):

_____

Did you sleep through the night? _____NO_____YES

If not, how many times was your sleep disrupted? _____

How many hours did you sleep during the night? _____

COMMENTS AND MORE INFORMATION: Make notes for and about visits with your healthcare provider, side effects from treatments you may be experiencing, any problems you are having coping with your pain, and more about some of your previous answers or questions.

_____

_____

_____

7

6 DAILY BODY PAIN DIAGRAM

Mark each place on the diagram where you have had pain today by placing an 'X', circling the location, or shading the area .

Describe the type of pain:

Shooting   Deep
Tingling   Sharp
Numbness   Burning / Hot
Cold   Aching
Surface Pain   Gnawing / Biting
Stabbing   Electrical / Shocks
Dull   Other_____
Stinging

COMMENTS AND MORE INFORMATION:

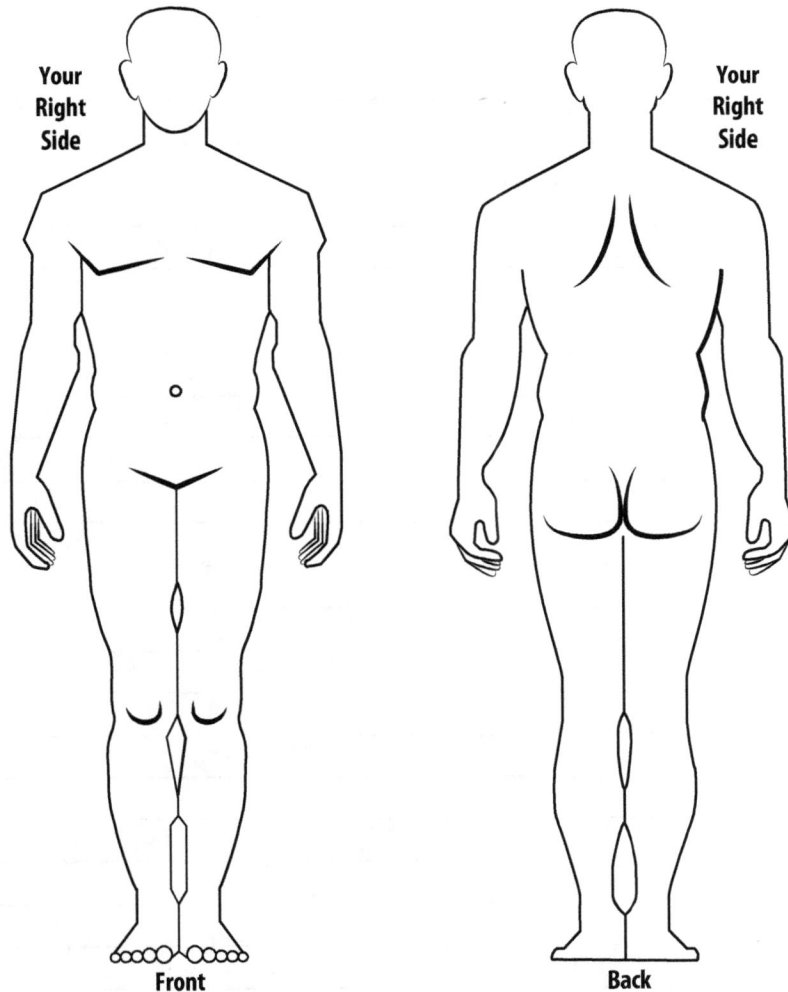

Your Right Side

Your Right Side

Front

Back

8

1 DAILY
TREATMENT PLAN

As you and your medical team develop new treatment plans, record your plan for the day including:
1.) New medications,
2.) Increases or decreases to medications,
3.) Exercises, physical therapy, or any other treatments,
4.) It will be especially helpful to record any side effects you experience as you add new treatments.
   This can help determine which types of treatments will work best for you.

Contact your care provider with any bad reactions or side effects to determine if you should discontinue the medication or treatment.

MEDICATION / TREATMENT	AMOUNT / TIME / COMMENTS

DAY_____ DATE_____ WEIGHT_____

INSTRUCTIONS:
1.) **Place an 'X'** on the chart below where the lines for the time of day and your level of pain meet.
2.) **Connect the points** on your DAILY PAIN CHART so your medical team can see when your status changed.
3.) **Refer to the EXAMPLES** in the front of this book for further direction.

2 DAILY PAIN CHART

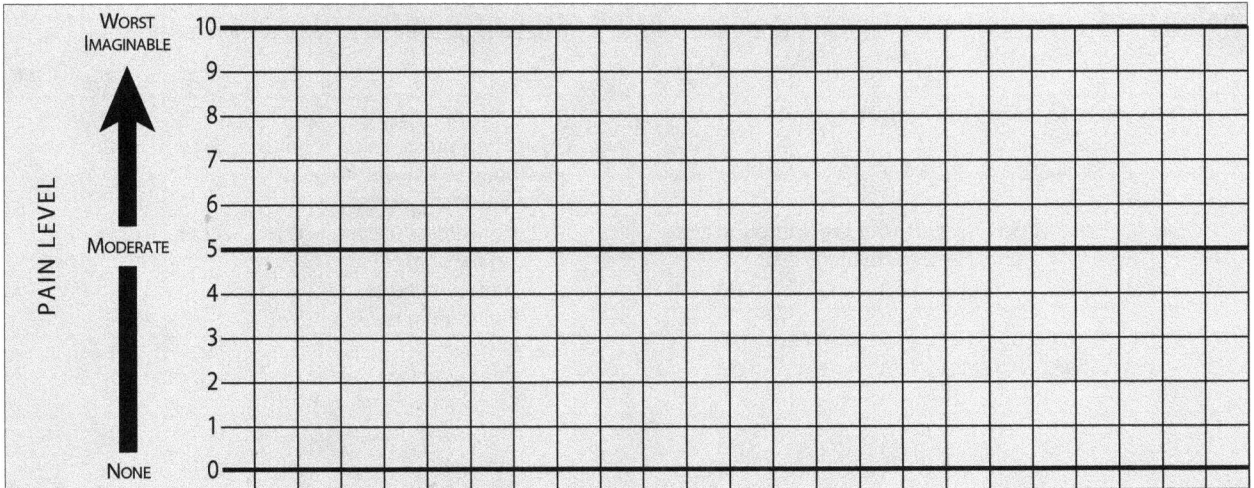

PAIN LEVEL

WORST IMAGINABLE	10
	9
	8
	7
	6
MODERATE	5
	4
	3
	2
	1
NONE	0

3 DAILY MEDICATION

MEDICINE NAME / DOSE

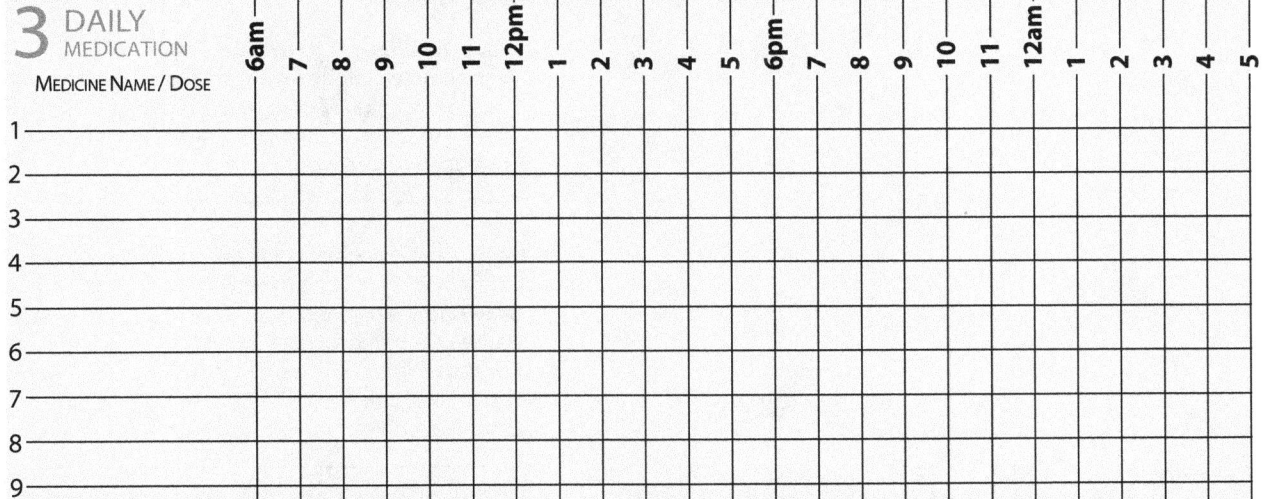

6am 7 8 9 10 11 12pm 1 2 3 4 5 6pm 7 8 9 10 11 12am 1 2 3 4 5

1
2
3
4
5
6
7
8
9

4 DAILY PHYSIOLOGY

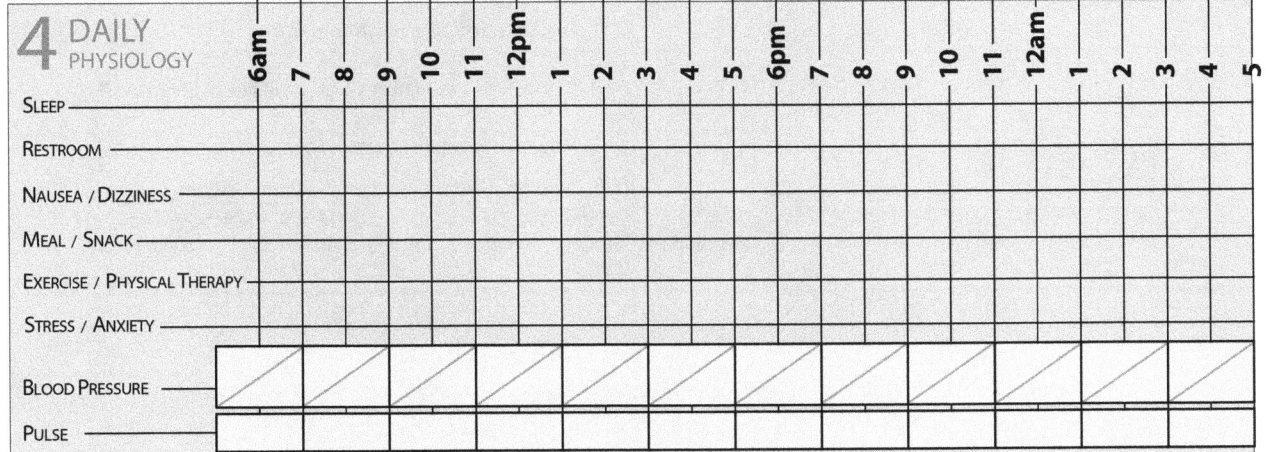

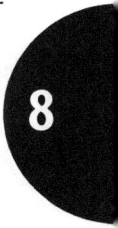

6am 7 8 9 10 11 12pm 1 2 3 4 5 6pm 7 8 9 10 11 12am 1 2 3 4 5

SLEEP
RESTROOM
NAUSEA / DIZZINESS
MEAL / SNACK
EXERCISE / PHYSICAL THERAPY
STRESS / ANXIETY
BLOOD PRESSURE
PULSE

5 DAILY
PAIN SUMMARY

Were there times during the day that you experienced unrelieved breakthrough pain? _____NO _____YES

How many times did this happen today?

1 2 3 4 5 6 7 8 9 10 more than 10

Did any specific activity start your breakthrough pain? _____NO _____YES: What activities?

_____

Put an "X" on the body diagram to show each place you've had **BREAKTHROUGH PAIN** today.

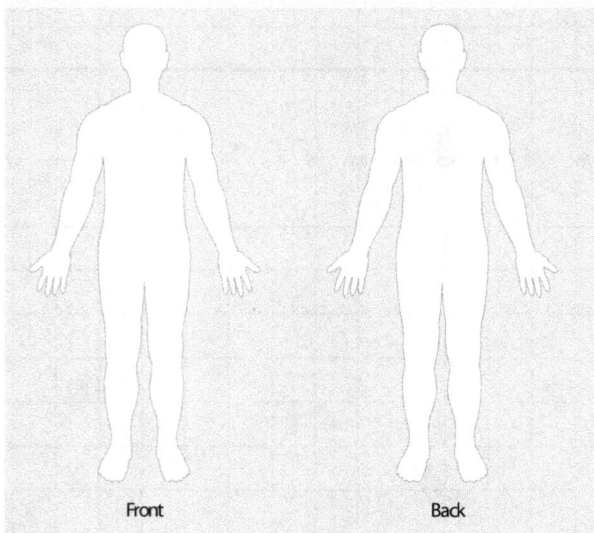

Front   Back

NON-DRUG THERAPIES
(other than prescription or other medicines)

_____
_____

ACTIVITIES/EXERCISE

_____

What was your average level of pain today?

0 1 2 3 4 5 6 7 8 9 10

Other than prescription medicine, did you do anything else today to relieve the pain? _____NO _____YES:
(Note any that you used.)
_____ Non-prescription drugs (e.g., acetaminophen, ibuprofen)
_____ Herbal remedies
_____ Hot or cold packs
_____ Exercise
_____ Changing position (such as lying down or elevating your legs)
_____ Physical therapy
_____ Massage
_____ Acupuncture
_____ Rest
_____ Prayer, meditation, guided imagery
_____ Relaxation technique (hypnosis, biofeedback)
_____ Creative technique (art or music therapy)
_____ Other (e.g., specific chiropractic manipulation, osteopathic treatments):

_____

Check any of these common side effects that you've noticed after taking your pain medicine:
_____ Drowsiness, sleepiness
_____ Nausea, vomiting, upset stomach
_____ Constipation
_____ Lack of appetite
_____ Other (describe):

_____

Did you sleep through the night? _____NO_____YES

If not, how many times was your sleep disrupted? _____

How many hours did you sleep during the night? _____

COMMENTS AND MORE INFORMATION: Make notes for and about visits with your healthcare provider, side effects from treatments you may be experiencing, any problems you are having coping with your pain, and more about some of your previous answers or questions.

_____
_____
_____

6 DAILY BODY PAIN DIAGRAM

Mark each place on the diagram where you have had pain today by placing an 'X', circling the location, or shading the area.

Describe the type of pain:

Shooting	Deep
Tingling	Sharp
Numbness	Burning / Hot
Cold	Aching
Surface Pain	Gnawing / Biting
Stabbing	Electrical / Shocks
Dull	Other_____
Stinging	

COMMENTS AND MORE INFORMATION:

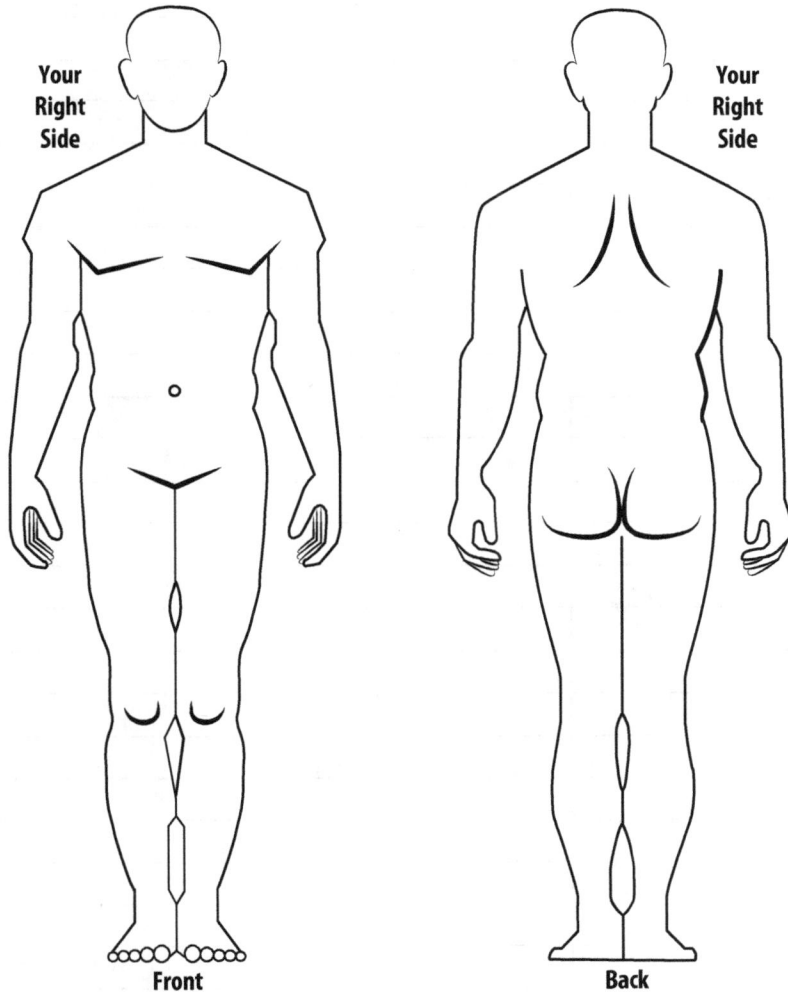

Your Right Side

Your Right Side

Front

Back

1 DAILY
TREATMENT PLAN

As you and your medical team develop new treatment plans, record your plan for the day including:
1.) New medications,
2.) Increases or decreases to medications,
3.) Exercises, physical therapy, or any other treatments,
4.) It will be especially helpful to record any side effects you experience as you add new treatments.
   This can help determine which types of treatments will work best for you.

Contact your care provider with any bad reactions or side effects to determine if you should discontinue the medication or treatment.

9

MEDICATION / TREATMENT	AMOUNT / TIME / COMMENTS

INSTRUCTIONS:

1.) **Place an 'X'** on the chart below where the lines for the time of day and your level of pain meet.
2.) **Connect the points** on your DAILY PAIN CHART so your medical team can see when your status changed.
3.) **Refer to the EXAMPLES** in the front of this book for further direction.

DAY_____ DATE_____ WEIGHT_____

2 DAILY PAIN CHART

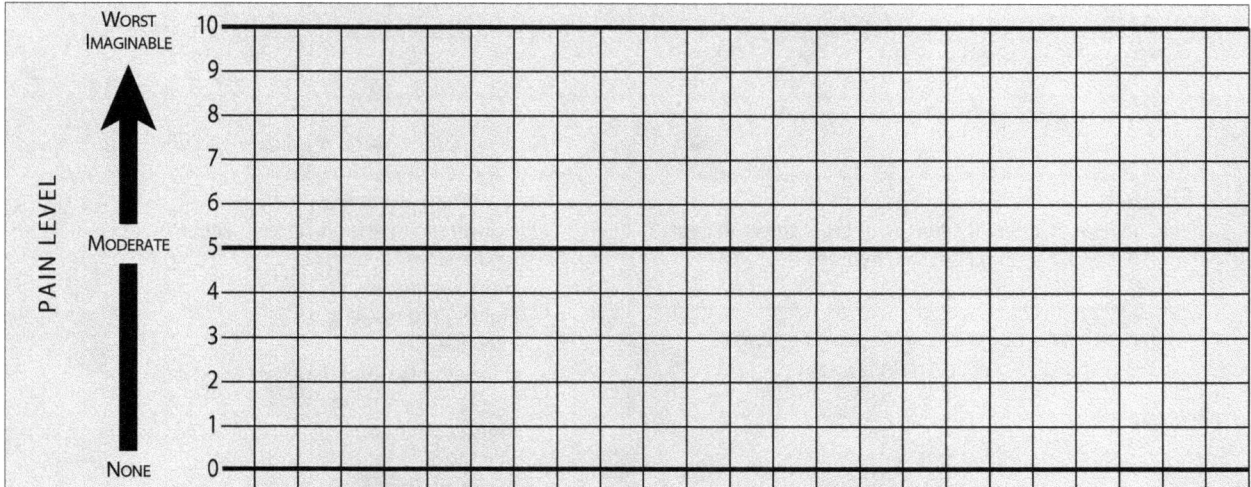

PAIN LEVEL

WORST IMAGINABLE	10
	9
	8
	7
	6
MODERATE	5
	4
	3
	2
	1
NONE	0

3 DAILY MEDICATION

MEDICINE NAME / DOSE

6am 7 8 9 10 11 12pm 1 2 3 4 5 6pm 7 8 9 10 11 12am 1 2 3 4 5

1
2
3
4
5
6
7
8
9

4 DAILY PHYSIOLOGY

6am 7 8 9 10 11 12pm 1 2 3 4 5 6pm 7 8 9 10 11 12am 1 2 3 4 5

SLEEP
RESTROOM
NAUSEA / DIZZINESS
MEAL / SNACK
EXERCISE / PHYSICAL THERAPY
STRESS / ANXIETY
BLOOD PRESSURE
PULSE

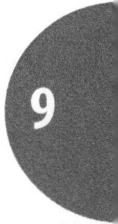

9

5 DAILY
PAIN SUMMARY

Were there times during the day that you experienced unrelieved breakthrough pain? _____NO _____YES

How many times did this happen today?

   1 2 3 4 5 6 7 8 9 10 more than 10

Did any specific activity start your breakthrough pain? _____NO _____YES: What activities?

_____

Put an "X" on the body diagram to show each place you've had **BREAKTHROUGH PAIN** today.

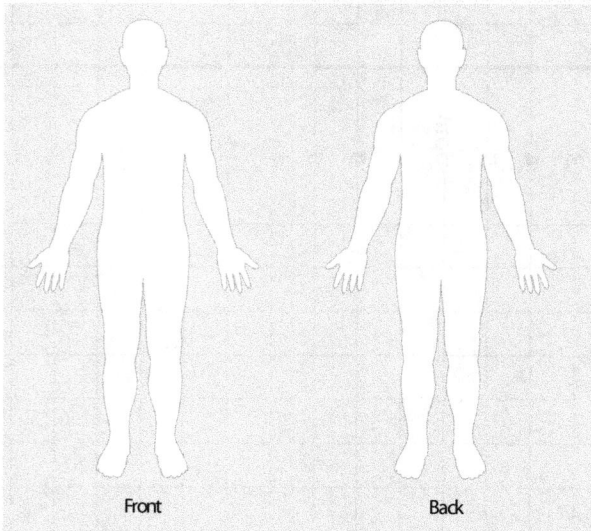

Front   Back

NON-DRUG THERAPIES
(other than prescription or other medicines)

_____

_____

ACTIVITIES/EXERCISE

_____

_____

What was your average level of pain today?

  0 1 2 3 4 5 6 7 8 9 10

Other than prescription medicine, did you do anything else today to relieve the pain? _____NO _____YES: (Note any that you used.)
_____ Non-prescription drugs (e.g., acetaminophen, ibuprofen)
_____ Herbal remedies
_____ Hot or cold packs
_____ Exercise
_____ Changing position (such as lying down or elevating your legs)
_____ Physical therapy
_____ Massage
_____ Acupuncture
_____ Rest
_____ Prayer, meditation, guided imagery
_____ Relaxation technique (hypnosis, biofeedback)
_____ Creative technique (art or music therapy)
_____ Other (e.g., specific chiropractic manipulation, osteopathic treatments):

_____

Check any of these common side effects that you've noticed after taking your pain medicine:
_____ Drowsiness, sleepiness
_____ Nausea, vomiting, upset stomach
_____ Constipation
_____ Lack of appetite
_____ Other (describe):

_____

Did you sleep through the night? _____NO_____YES

If not, how many times was your sleep disrupted? _____

How many hours did you sleep during the night? _____

COMMENTS AND MORE INFORMATION: Make notes for and about visits with your healthcare provider, side effects from treatments you may be experiencing, any problems you are having coping with your pain, and more about some of your previous answers or questions.

_____

_____

_____

6 DAILY BODY PAIN DIAGRAM

Mark each place on the diagram where you have had pain today by placing an 'X', circling the location, or shading the area .

Describe the type of pain:

Shooting	Deep
Tingling	Sharp
Numbness	Burning / Hot
Cold	Aching
Surface Pain	Gnawing / Biting
Stabbing	Electrical / Shocks
Dull	Other_____
Stinging	

COMMENTS AND MORE INFORMATION:

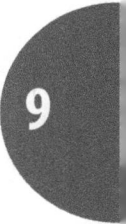

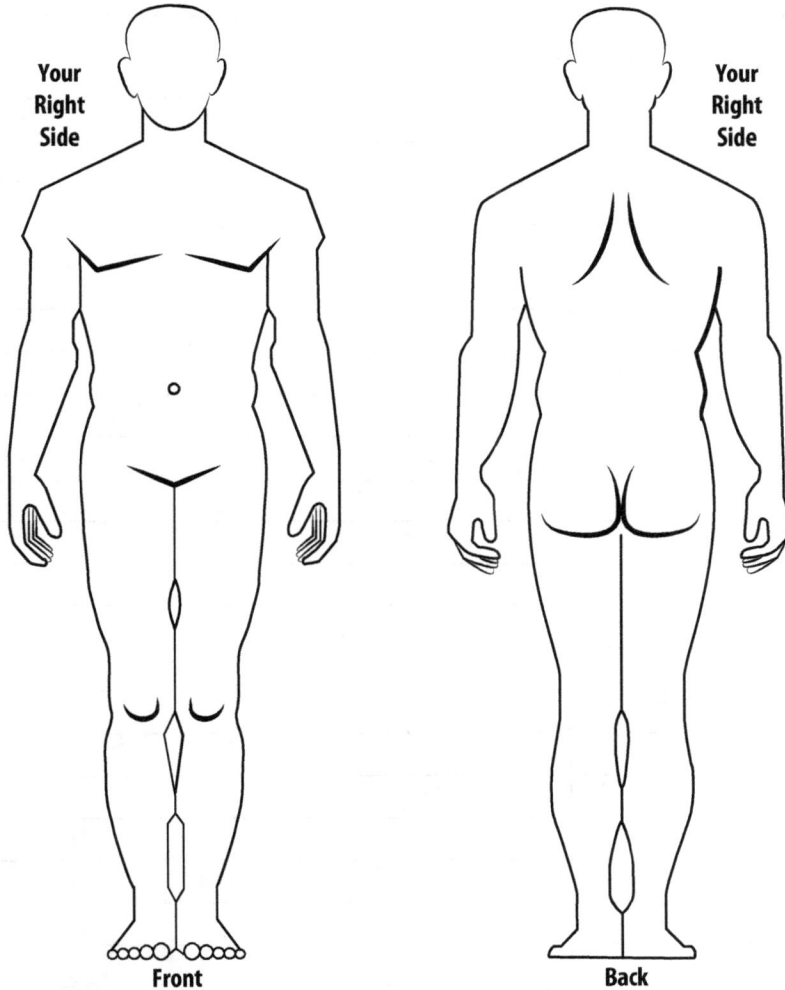

9

Your Right Side

Your Right Side

Front

Back

1 DAILY
TREATMENT PLAN

As you and your medical team develop new treatment plans, record your plan for the day including:
1.) New medications,
2.) Increases or decreases to medications,
3.) Exercises, physical therapy, or any other treatments,
4.) It will be especially helpful to record any side effects you experience as you add new treatments.
   This can help determine which types of treatments will work best for you.

Contact your care provider with any bad reactions or side effects to determine if you should discontinue the medication or treatment.

10

MEDICATION / TREATMENT	AMOUNT / TIME / COMMENTS

DAY_____ DATE_____ WEIGHT_____

INSTRUCTIONS:
1.) **Place an 'X'** on the chart below where the lines for the time of day and your level of pain meet.
2.) **Connect the points** on your DAILY PAIN CHART so your medical team can see when your status changed.
3.) **Refer to the EXAMPLES** in the front of this book for further direction.

2 DAILY PAIN CHART

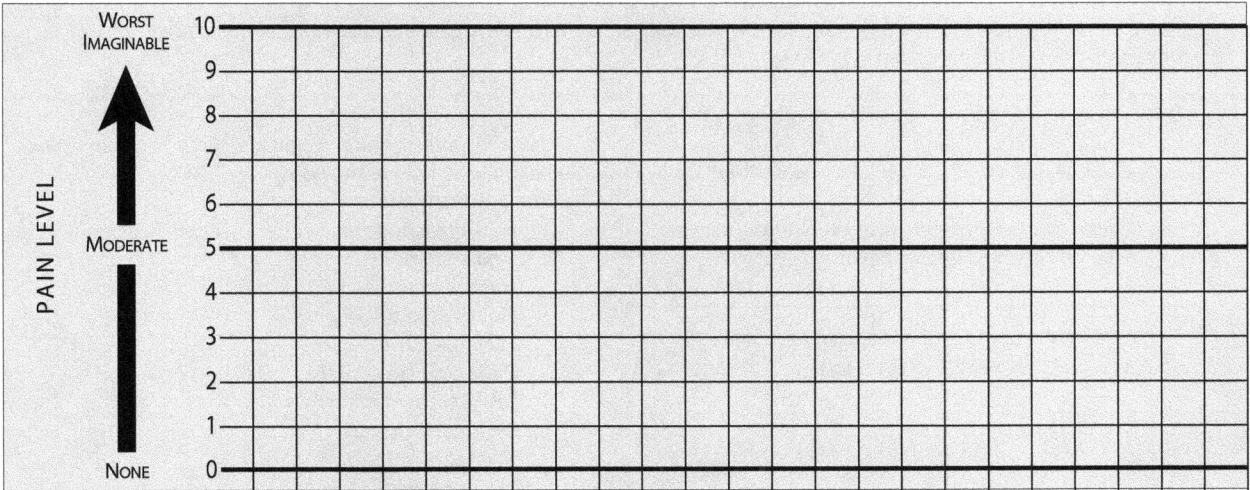

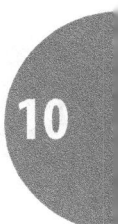

3 DAILY MEDICATION

MEDICINE NAME / DOSE

	6am	7	8	9	10	11	12pm	1	2	3	4	5	6pm	7	8	9	10	11	12am	1	2	3	4	5
1																								
2																								
3																								
4																								
5																								
6																								
7																								
8																								
9																								

4 DAILY PHYSIOLOGY

	6am	7	8	9	10	11	12pm	1	2	3	4	5	6pm	7	8	9	10	11	12am	1	2	3	4	5
SLEEP																								
RESTROOM																								
NAUSEA / DIZZINESS																								
MEAL / SNACK																								
EXERCISE / PHYSICAL THERAPY																								
STRESS / ANXIETY																								
BLOOD PRESSURE																								
PULSE																								

5 DAILY
PAIN SUMMARY

Were there times during the day that you experienced unrelieved breakthrough pain? ____NO ____YES

How many times did this happen today?

1 2 3 4 5 6 7 8 9 10 more than 10

Did any specific activity start your breakthrough pain? ____NO ____YES: What activities?

_____

Put an "X" on the body diagram to show each place you've had **BREAKTHROUGH PAIN** today.

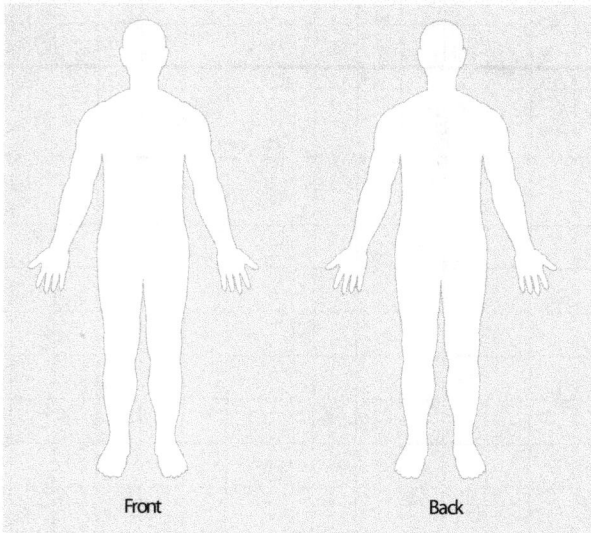

Front   Back

NON-DRUG THERAPIES
(other than prescription or other medicines)

_____

_____

ACTIVITIES/EXERCISE

_____

What was your average level of pain today?

0 1 2 3 4 5 6 7 8 9 10

Other than prescription medicine, did you do anything else today to relieve the pain? ____NO ____YES:
(Note any that you used.)
____ Non-prescription drugs (e.g., acetaminophen, ibuprofen)
____ Herbal remedies
____ Hot or cold packs
____ Exercise
____ Changing position (such as lying down or elevating your legs)
____ Physical therapy
____ Massage
____ Acupuncture
____ Rest
____ Prayer, meditation, guided imagery
____ Relaxation technique (hypnosis, biofeedback)
____ Creative technique (art or music therapy)
____ Other (e.g., specific chiropractic manipulation, osteopathic treatments):

_____

Check any of these common side effects that you've noticed after taking your pain medicine:
____ Drowsiness, sleepiness
____ Nausea, vomiting, upset stomach
____ Constipation
____ Lack of appetite
____ Other (describe):

_____

Did you sleep through the night? ____NO____YES

If not, how many times was your sleep disrupted? _____

How many hours did you sleep during the night? _____

COMMENTS AND MORE INFORMATION: Make notes for and about visits with your healthcare provider, side effects from treatments you may be experiencing, any problems you are having coping with your pain, and more about some of your previous answers or questions.

_____

_____

6 DAILY BODY PAIN DIAGRAM

Mark each place on the diagram where you have had pain today by placing an 'X', circling the location, or shading the area .

Describe the type of pain:

Shooting
Tingling
Numbness
Cold
Surface Pain
Stabbing
Dull
Stinging

Deep
Sharp
Burning / Hot
Aching
Gnawing / Biting
Electrical / Shocks
Other_____

COMMENTS AND MORE INFORMATION:

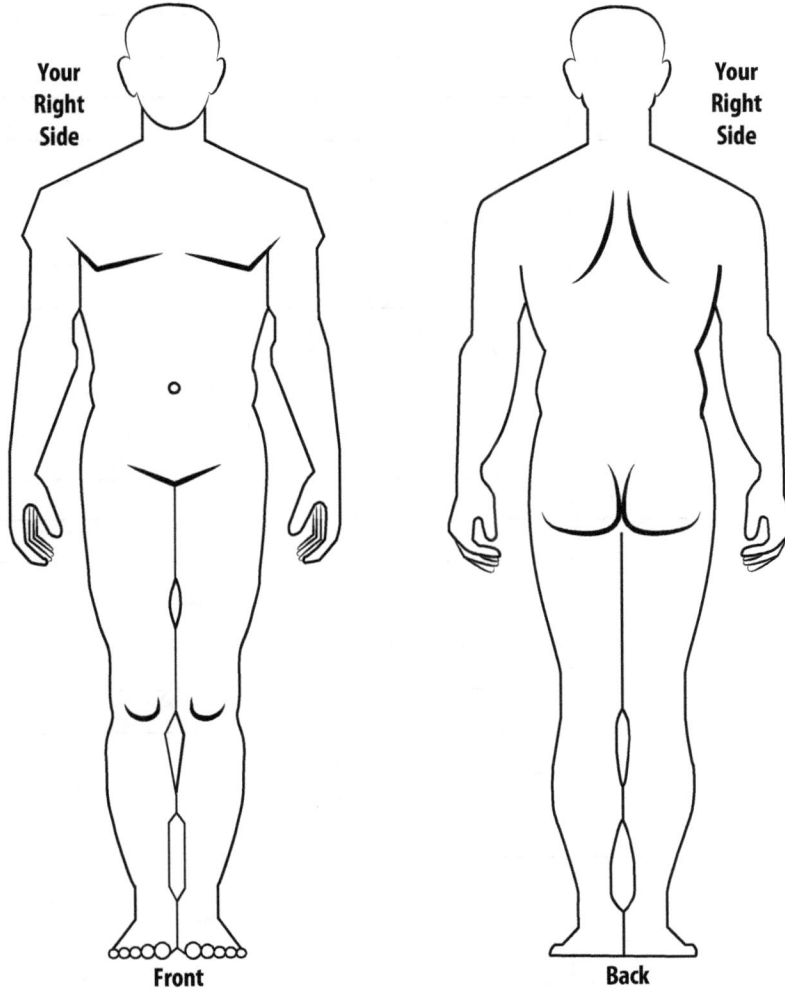

10

Your
Right
Side

Your
Right
Side

Front

Back

1 DAILY
TREATMENT PLAN

As you and your medical team develop new treatment plans, record your plan for the day including:
1.) New medications,
2.) Increases or decreases to medications,
3.) Exercises, physical therapy, or any other treatments,
4.) It will be especially helpful to record any side effects you experience as you add new treatments.
   This can help determine which types of treatments will work best for you.

Contact your care provider with any bad reactions or side effects to determine if you should discontinue the medication or treatment.

MEDICATION / TREATMENT	AMOUNT / TIME / COMMENTS

11

DAY_____ DATE_____ WEIGHT_____

INSTRUCTIONS:
1.) **Place an 'X'** on the chart below where the lines for the time of day and your level of pain meet.
2.) **Connect the points** on your DAILY PAIN CHART so your medical team can see when your status changed.
3.) **Refer to the EXAMPLES** in the front of this book for further direction.

2 DAILY PAIN CHART

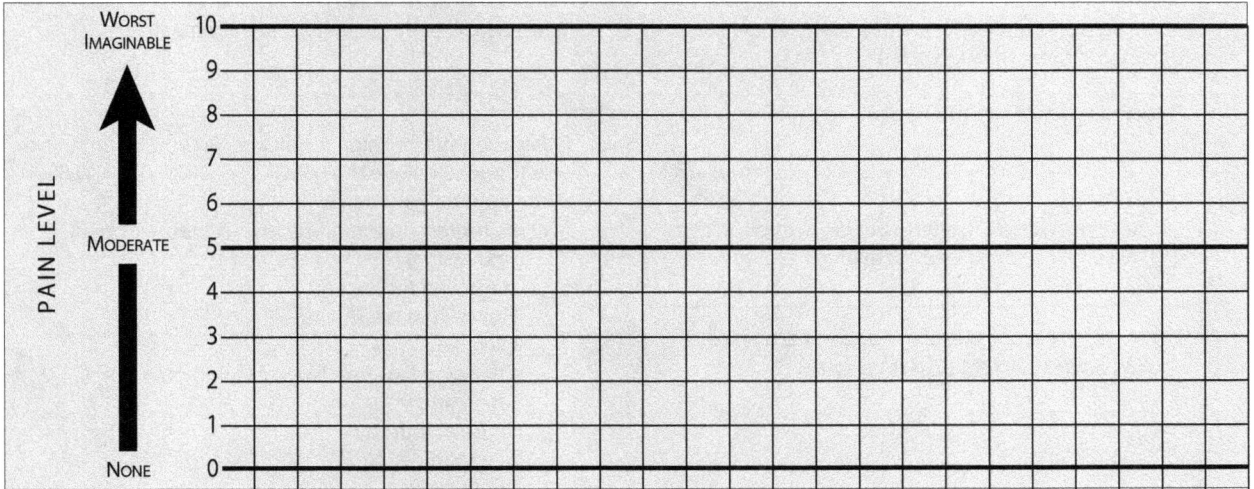

3 DAILY MEDICATION

MEDICINE NAME / DOSE

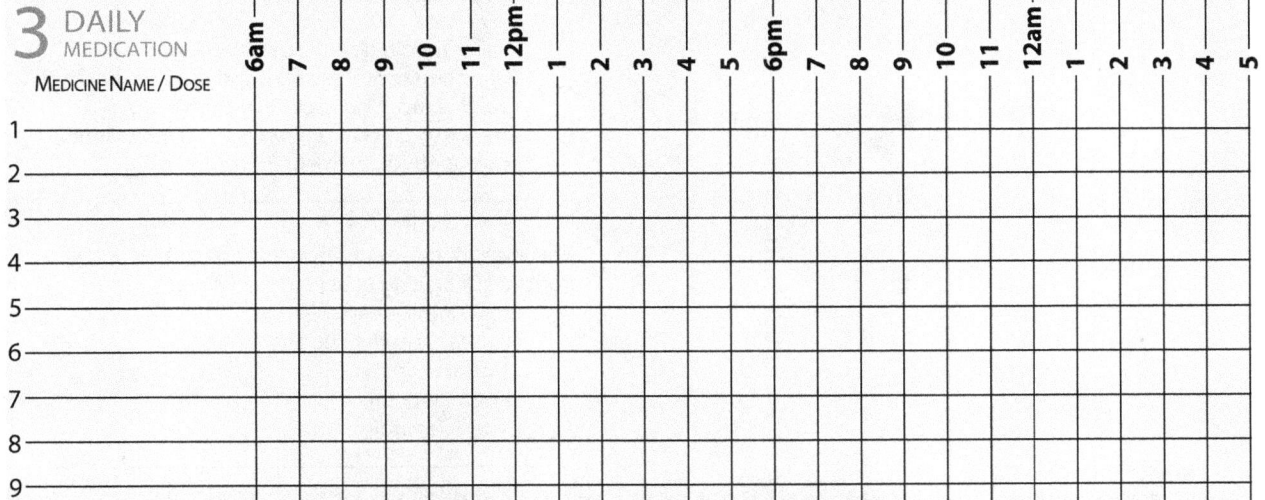

4 DAILY PHYSIOLOGY

SLEEP
RESTROOM
NAUSEA / DIZZINESS
MEAL / SNACK
EXERCISE / PHYSICAL THERAPY
STRESS / ANXIETY
BLOOD PRESSURE
PULSE

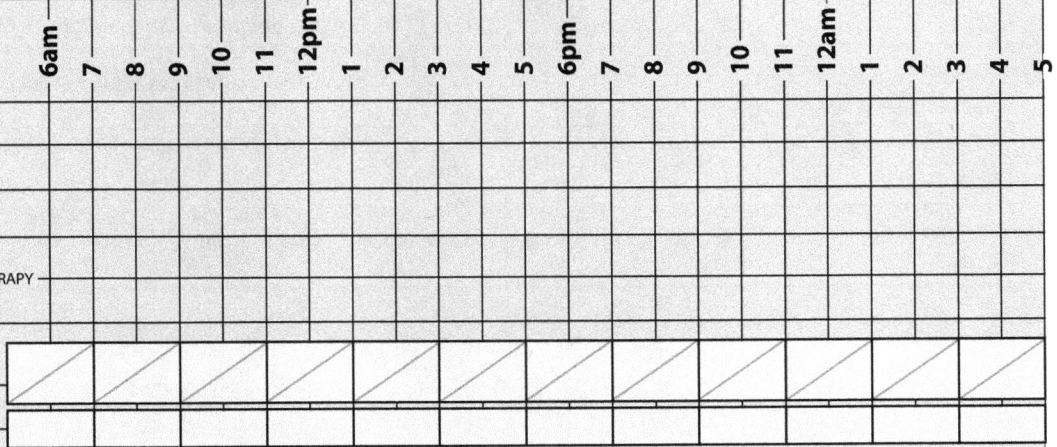

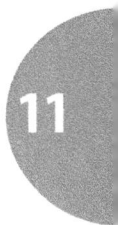

5 DAILY
PAIN SUMMARY

Were there times during the day that you experienced unrelieved breakthrough pain? ____NO ____YES

How many times did this happen today?

    1 2 3 4 5 6 7 8 9 10 more than 10

Did any specific activity start your breakthrough pain? ____NO ____YES: What activities?

_____

Put an "X" on the body diagram to show each place you've had **BREAKTHROUGH PAIN** today.

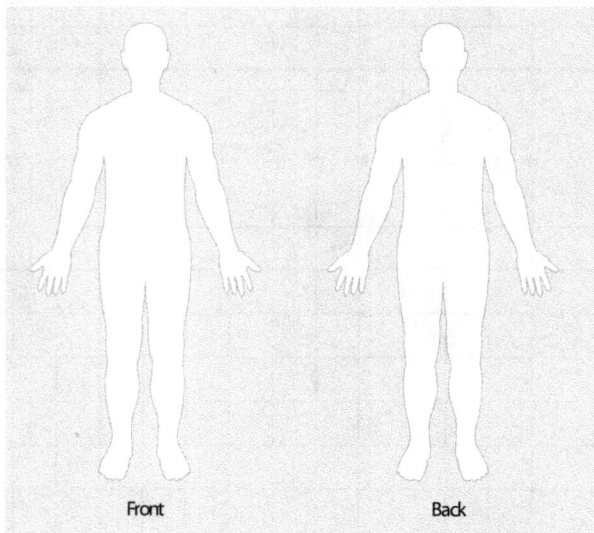

Front   Back

NON-DRUG THERAPIES
(other than prescription or other medicines)

_____

_____

ACTIVITIES/EXERCISE

_____

What was your average level of pain today?

  0 1 2 3 4 5 6 7 8 9 10

Other than prescription medicine, did you do anything else today to relieve the pain? ____NO ____YES: (Note any that you used.)
____ Non-prescription drugs (e.g., acetaminophen, ibuprofen)
____ Herbal remedies
____ Hot or cold packs
____ Exercise
____ Changing position (such as lying down or elevating your legs)
____ Physical therapy
____ Massage
____ Acupuncture
____ Rest
____ Prayer, meditation, guided imagery
____ Relaxation technique (hypnosis, biofeedback)
____ Creative technique (art or music therapy)
____ Other (e.g., specific chiropractic manipulation, osteopathic treatments):

_____

Check any of these common side effects that you've noticed after taking your pain medicine:
____ Drowsiness, sleepiness
____ Nausea, vomiting, upset stomach
____ Constipation
____ Lack of appetite
____ Other (describe):

_____

Did you sleep through the night? ____NO____YES

If not, how many times was your sleep disrupted? _____

How many hours did you sleep during the night? _____

COMMENTS AND MORE INFORMATION: Make notes for and about visits with your healthcare provider, side effects from treatments you may be experiencing, any problems you are having coping with your pain, and more about some of your previous answers or questions.

_____

_____

_____

6 DAILY BODY PAIN DIAGRAM

Mark each place on the diagram where you have had pain today by placing an 'X', circling the location, or shading the area .

Describe the type of pain:

Shooting	Deep
Tingling	Sharp
Numbness	Burning / Hot
Cold	Aching
Surface Pain	Gnawing / Biting
Stabbing	Electrical / Shocks
Dull	Other_____
Stinging	

COMMENTS AND MORE INFORMATION:

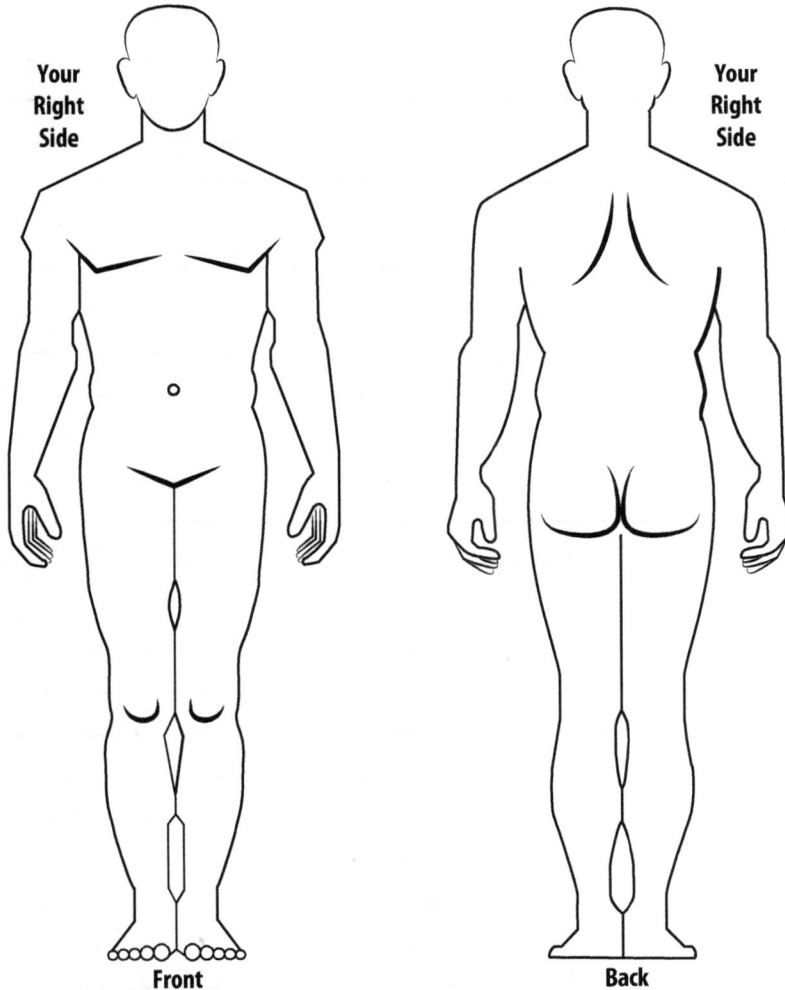

Your Right Side

Your Right Side

Front

Back

11

1 DAILY
TREATMENT PLAN

As you and your medical team develop new treatment plans, record your plan for the day including:

1.) New medications,
2.) Increases or decreases to medications,
3.) Exercises, physical therapy, or any other treatments,
4.) It will be especially helpful to record any side effects you experience as you add new treatments. This can help determine which types of treatments will work best for you.

Contact your care provider with any bad reactions or side effects to determine if you should discontinue the medication or treatment.

MEDICATION / TREATMENT	AMOUNT / TIME / COMMENTS

12

DAY_____ DATE_____ WEIGHT_____

INSTRUCTIONS:
1.) **Place an 'X'** on the chart below where the lines for the time of day and your level of pain meet.
2.) **Connect the points** on your DAILY PAIN CHART so your medical team can see when your status changed.
3.) **Refer to the EXAMPLES** in the front of this book for further direction.

2 DAILY PAIN CHART

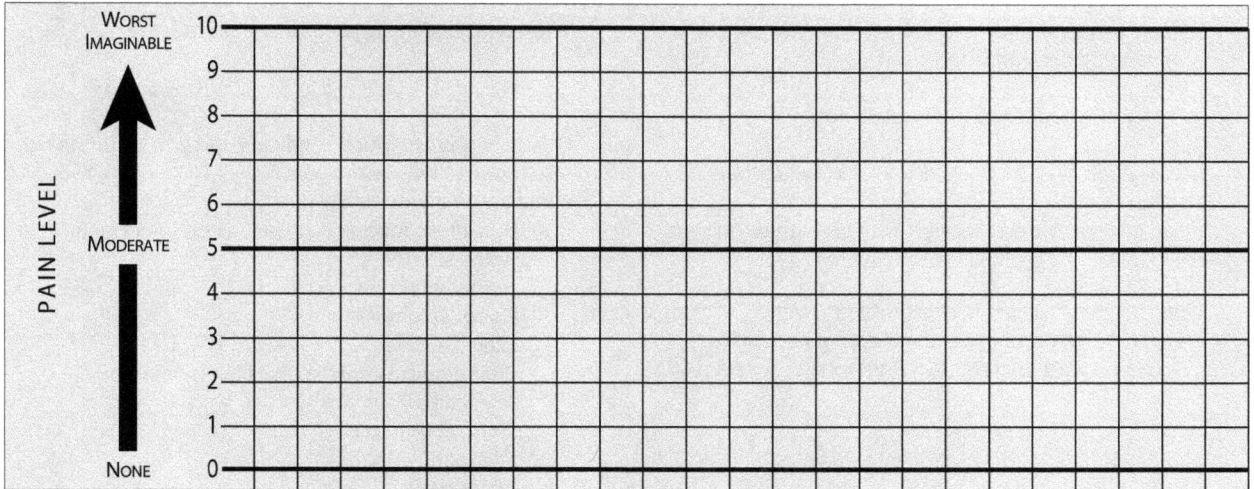

PAIN LEVEL

WORST IMAGINABLE — 10
9
8
7
6
MODERATE — 5
4
3
2
1
NONE — 0

3 DAILY MEDICATION

MEDICINE NAME / DOSE

6am 7 8 9 10 11 12pm 1 2 3 4 5 6pm 7 8 9 10 11 12am 1 2 3 4 5

1
2
3
4
5
6
7
8
9

4 DAILY PHYSIOLOGY

6am 7 8 9 10 11 12pm 1 2 3 4 5 6pm 7 8 9 10 11 12am 1 2 3 4 5

SLEEP
RESTROOM
NAUSEA / DIZZINESS
MEAL / SNACK
EXERCISE / PHYSICAL THERAPY
STRESS / ANXIETY
BLOOD PRESSURE
PULSE

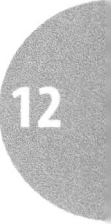

12

5 DAILY
PAIN SUMMARY

Were there times during the day that you experienced unrelieved breakthrough pain? ____NO ____YES

How many times did this happen today?

1 2 3 4 5 6 7 8 9 10 more than 10

Did any specific activity start your breakthrough pain?
____NO ____YES: What activities?

_____

Put an "X" on the body diagram to show each place you've had **BREAKTHROUGH PAIN** today.

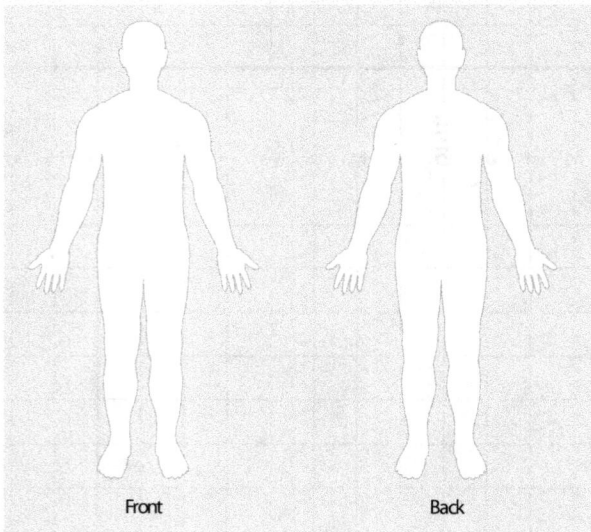

Front   Back

NON-DRUG THERAPIES
(other than prescription or other medicines)

_____

_____

ACTIVITIES/EXERCISE

_____

What was your average level of pain today?

0 1 2 3 4 5 6 7 8 9 10

Other than prescription medicine, did you do anything else today to relieve the pain? ____NO ____YES:
(Note any that you used.)
____ Non-prescription drugs (e.g., acetaminophen, ibuprofen)
____ Herbal remedies
____ Hot or cold packs
____ Exercise
____ Changing position (such as lying down or elevating your legs)
____ Physical therapy
____ Massage
____ Acupuncture
____ Rest
____ Prayer, meditation, guided imagery
____ Relaxation technique (hypnosis, biofeedback)
____ Creative technique (art or music therapy)
____ Other (e.g., specific chiropractic manipulation, osteopathic treatments):

_____

Check any of these common side effects that you've noticed after taking your pain medicine:
____ Drowsiness, sleepiness
____ Nausea, vomiting, upset stomach
____ Constipation
____ Lack of appetite
____ Other (describe):

_____

Did you sleep through the night? ____NO____YES

If not, how many times was your sleep disrupted? _____

How many hours did you sleep during the night? _____

COMMENTS AND MORE INFORMATION: Make notes for and about visits with your healthcare provider, side effects from treatments you may be experiencing, any problems you are having coping with your pain, and more about some of your previous answers or questions.

_____

_____

_____

12

6 DAILY BODY PAIN DIAGRAM

Mark each place on the diagram where you have had pain today by placing an 'X', circling the location, or shading the area .

Describe the type of pain:

Shooting	Deep
Tingling	Sharp
Numbness	Burning / Hot
Cold	Aching
Surface Pain	Gnawing / Biting
Stabbing	Electrical / Shocks
Dull	Other_____
Stinging	

COMMENTS AND MORE INFORMATION:

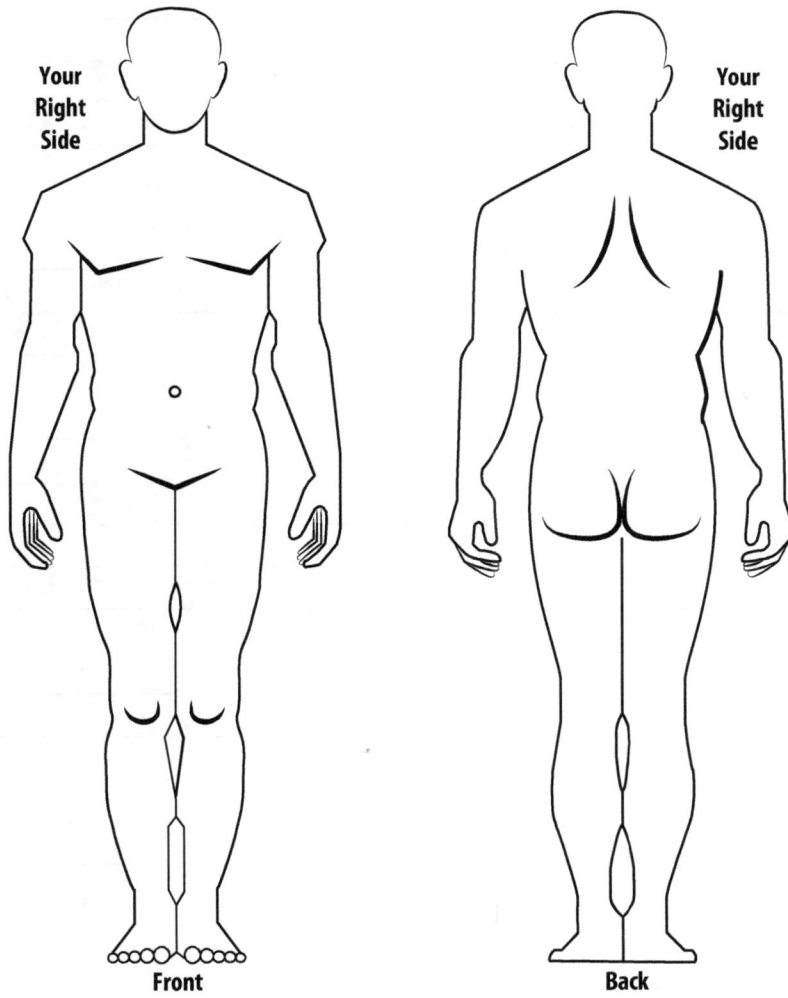

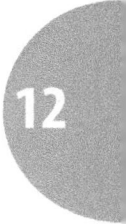

Your Right Side

Your Right Side

Front

Back

12

1 DAILY
TREATMENT PLAN

As you and your medical team develop new treatment plans, record your plan for the day including:
1.) New medications,
2.) Increases or decreases to medications,
3.) Exercises, physical therapy, or any other treatments,
4.) It will be especially helpful to record any side effects you experience as you add new treatments.
   This can help determine which types of treatments will work best for you.

Contact your care provider with any bad reactions or side effects to determine if you should discontinue the medication or treatment.

MEDICATION / TREATMENT	AMOUNT / TIME / COMMENTS

13

INSTRUCTIONS:
1.) **Place an 'X'** on the chart below where the lines for the time of day and your level of pain meet.
2.) **Connect the points** on your DAILY PAIN CHART so your medical team can see when your status changed.
3.) **Refer to the EXAMPLES** in the front of this book for further direction.

DAY_____ DATE_____ WEIGHT_____

2 DAILY PAIN CHART

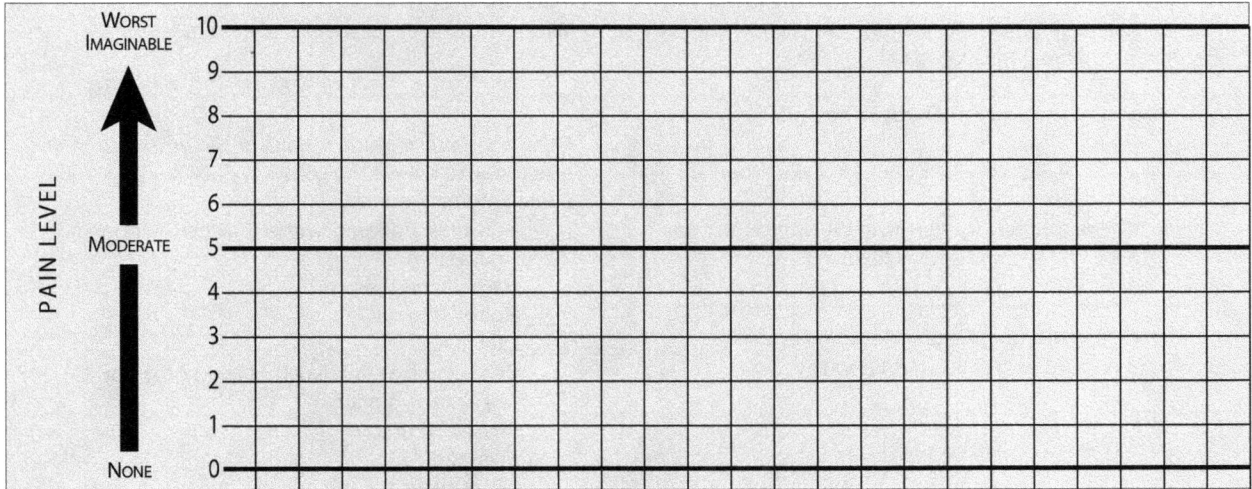

PAIN LEVEL

WORST IMAGINABLE — 10
9
8
7
6
MODERATE — 5
4
3
2
1
NONE — 0

3 DAILY MEDICATION

MEDICINE NAME / DOSE

6am 7 8 9 10 11 12pm 1 2 3 4 5 6pm 7 8 9 10 11 12am 1 2 3 4 5

1
2
3
4
5
6
7
8
9

4 DAILY PHYSIOLOGY

6am 7 8 9 10 11 12pm 1 2 3 4 5 6pm 7 8 9 10 11 12am 1 2 3 4 5

SLEEP
RESTROOM
NAUSEA / DIZZINESS
MEAL / SNACK
EXERCISE / PHYSICAL THERAPY
STRESS / ANXIETY
BLOOD PRESSURE
PULSE

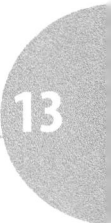

13

5 DAILY
PAIN SUMMARY

Were there times during the day that you experienced unrelieved breakthrough pain? ____NO ____YES

How many times did this happen today?

1 2 3 4 5 6 7 8 9 10 more than 10

Did any specific activity start your breakthrough pain?
____NO ____YES: What activities?

_____

Put an "X" on the body diagram to show each place you've had **BREAKTHROUGH PAIN** today.

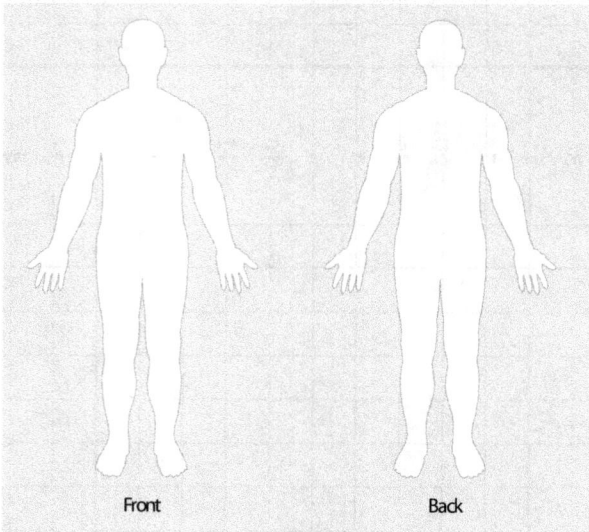

Front   Back

NON-DRUG THERAPIES
(other than prescription or other medicines)

_____

_____

ACTIVITIES/EXERCISE

_____

_____

What was your average level of pain today?

0 1 2 3 4 5 6 7 8 9 10

Other than prescription medicine, did you do anything else today to relieve the pain? ____NO ____YES:
(Note any that you used.)
____ Non-prescription drugs (e.g., acetaminophen, ibuprofen)
____ Herbal remedies
____ Hot or cold packs
____ Exercise
____ Changing position (such as lying down or elevating your legs)
____ Physical therapy
____ Massage
____ Acupuncture
____ Rest
____ Prayer, meditation, guided imagery
____ Relaxation technique (hypnosis, biofeedback)
____ Creative technique (art or music therapy)
____ Other (e.g., specific chiropractic manipulation, osteopathic treatments):

_____

Check any of these common side effects that you've noticed after taking your pain medicine:
____ Drowsiness, sleepiness
____ Nausea, vomiting, upset stomach
____ Constipation
____ Lack of appetite
____ Other (describe):

_____

Did you sleep through the night? ____NO____YES

If not, how many times was your sleep disrupted? _____

How many hours did you sleep during the night? _____

COMMENTS AND MORE INFORMATION: Make notes for and about visits with your healthcare provider, side effects from treatments you may be experiencing, any problems you are having coping with your pain, and more about some of your previous answers or questions.

_____

_____

_____

13

6 DAILY BODY PAIN DIAGRAM

Mark each place on the diagram where you have had pain today by placing an 'X', circling the location, or shading the area .

Describe the type of pain:

Shooting	Deep
Tingling	Sharp
Numbness	Burning / Hot
Cold	Aching
Surface Pain	Gnawing / Biting
Stabbing	Electrical / Shocks
Dull	Other_____
Stinging	

COMMENTS AND MORE INFORMATION:

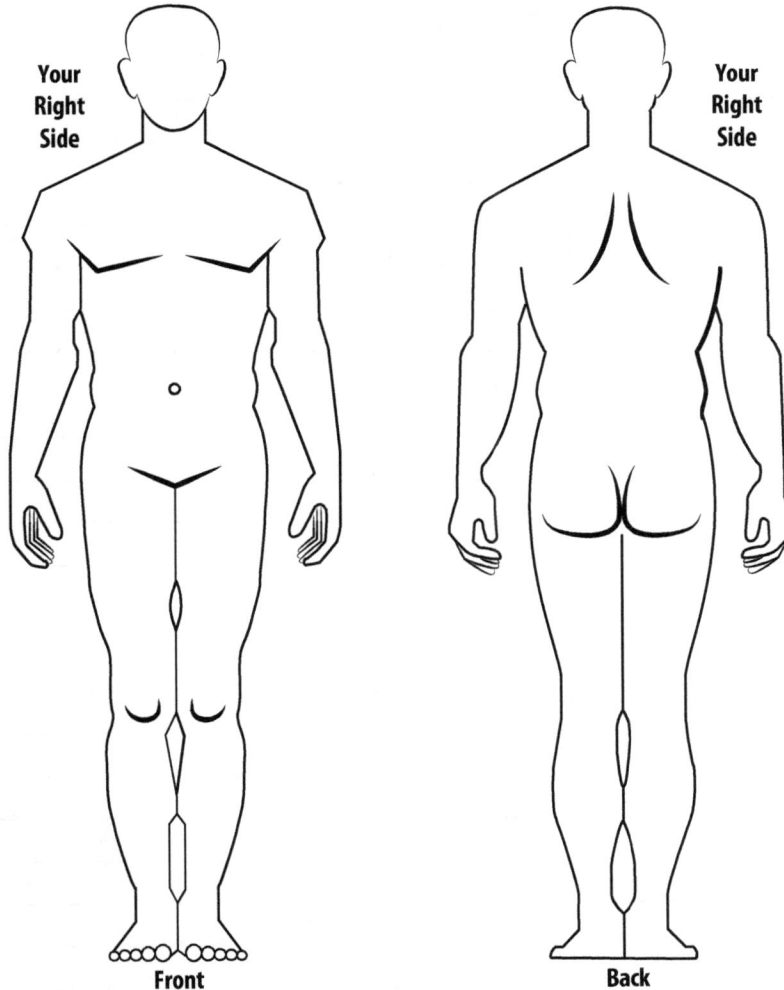

Your Right Side

Your Right Side

Front

Back

13

1 DAILY
TREATMENT PLAN

As you and your medical team develop new treatment plans, record your plan for the day including:
1.) New medications,
2.) Increases or decreases to medications,
3.) Exercises, physical therapy, or any other treatments,
4.) It will be especially helpful to record any side effects you experience as you add new treatments.
   This can help determine which types of treatments will work best for you.

Contact your care provider with any bad reactions or side effects to determine if you should discontinue
the medication or treatment.

MEDICATION / TREATMENT	AMOUNT / TIME / COMMENTS

14

DAY_____ DATE_____ WEIGHT_____

INSTRUCTIONS:
1.) **Place an 'X'** on the chart below where the lines for the time of day and your level of pain meet.
2.) **Connect the points** on your DAILY PAIN CHART so your medical team can see when your status changed.
3.) **Refer to the EXAMPLES** in the front of this book for further direction.

2 DAILY PAIN CHART

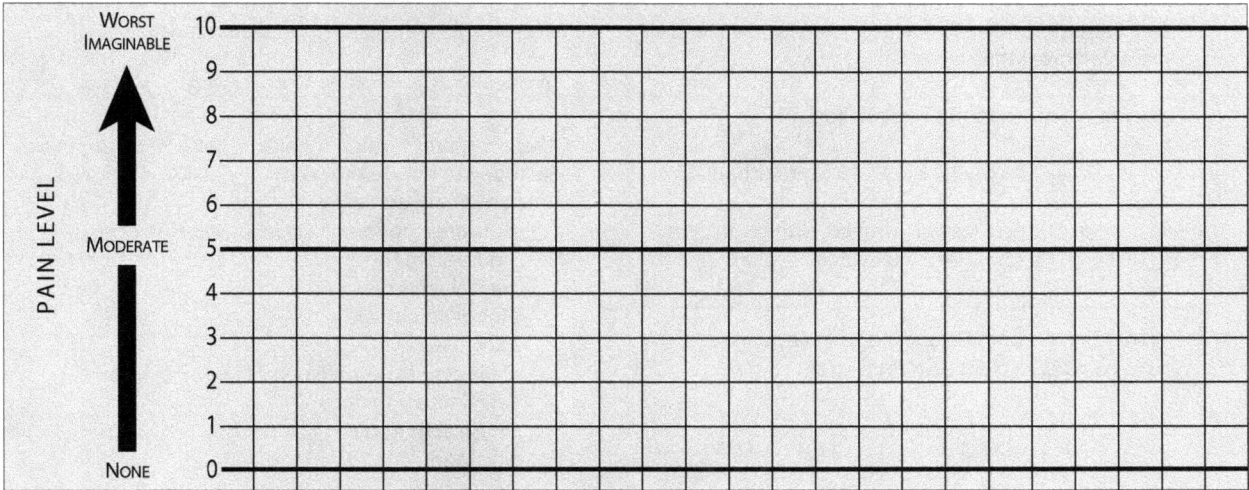

PAIN LEVEL

WORST IMAGINABLE	10
	9
	8
	7
	6
MODERATE	5
	4
	3
	2
	1
NONE	0

3 DAILY MEDICATION

MEDICINE NAME / DOSE

6am 7 8 9 10 11 12pm 1 2 3 4 5 6pm 7 8 9 10 11 12am 1 2 3 4 5

1
2
3
4
5
6
7
8
9

4 DAILY PHYSIOLOGY

6am 7 8 9 10 11 12pm 1 2 3 4 5 6pm 7 8 9 10 11 12am 1 2 3 4 5

SLEEP
RESTROOM
NAUSEA / DIZZINESS
MEAL / SNACK
EXERCISE / PHYSICAL THERAPY
STRESS / ANXIETY
BLOOD PRESSURE
PULSE

14

5 DAILY
PAIN SUMMARY

Were there times during the day that you experienced unrelieved breakthrough pain? ____NO ____YES

How many times did this happen today?

1 2 3 4 5 6 7 8 9 10 more than 10

Did any specific activity start your breakthrough pain? ____NO ____YES: What activities?

_____

Put an "X" on the body diagram to show each place you've had **BREAKTHROUGH PAIN** today.

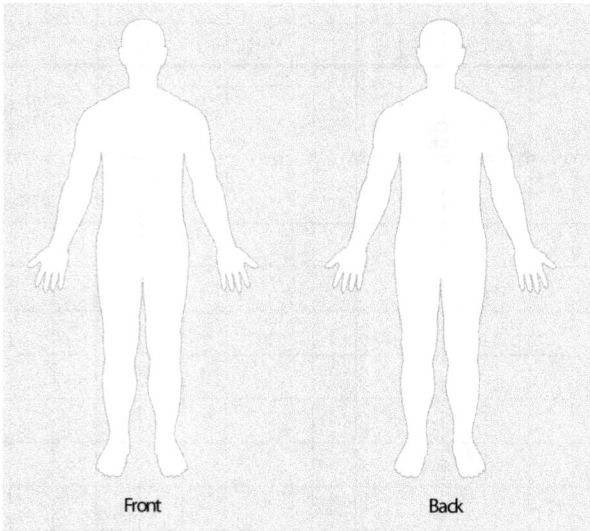

Front   Back

NON-DRUG THERAPIES
(other than prescription or other medicines)

_____

ACTIVITIES/EXERCISE

_____

What was your average level of pain today?

0 1 2 3 4 5 6 7 8 9 10

Other than prescription medicine, did you do anything else today to relieve the pain? ____NO ____YES: (Note any that you used.)
____ Non-prescription drugs (e.g., acetaminophen, ibuprofen)
____ Herbal remedies
____ Hot or cold packs
____ Exercise
____ Changing position (such as lying down or elevating your legs)
____ Physical therapy
____ Massage
____ Acupuncture
____ Rest
____ Prayer, meditation, guided imagery
____ Relaxation technique (hypnosis, biofeedback)
____ Creative technique (art or music therapy)
____ Other (e.g., specific chiropractic manipulation, osteopathic treatments):

_____

Check any of these common side effects that you've noticed after taking your pain medicine:
____ Drowsiness, sleepiness
____ Nausea, vomiting, upset stomach
____ Constipation
____ Lack of appetite
____ Other (describe):

_____

Did you sleep through the night? ____NO____YES

If not, how many times was your sleep disrupted? _____

How many hours did you sleep during the night? _____

COMMENTS AND MORE INFORMATION: Make notes for and about visits with your healthcare provider, side effects from treatments you may be experiencing, any problems you are having coping with your pain, and more about some of your previous answers or questions.

14

6 DAILY BODY PAIN DIAGRAM

Mark each place on the diagram where you have had pain today by placing an 'X', circling the location, or shading the area .

Describe the type of pain:

Shooting   Deep
Tingling   Sharp
Numbness   Burning / Hot
Cold   Aching
Surface Pain   Gnawing / Biting
Stabbing   Electrical / Shocks
Dull   Other_____
Stinging

COMMENTS AND MORE INFORMATION:

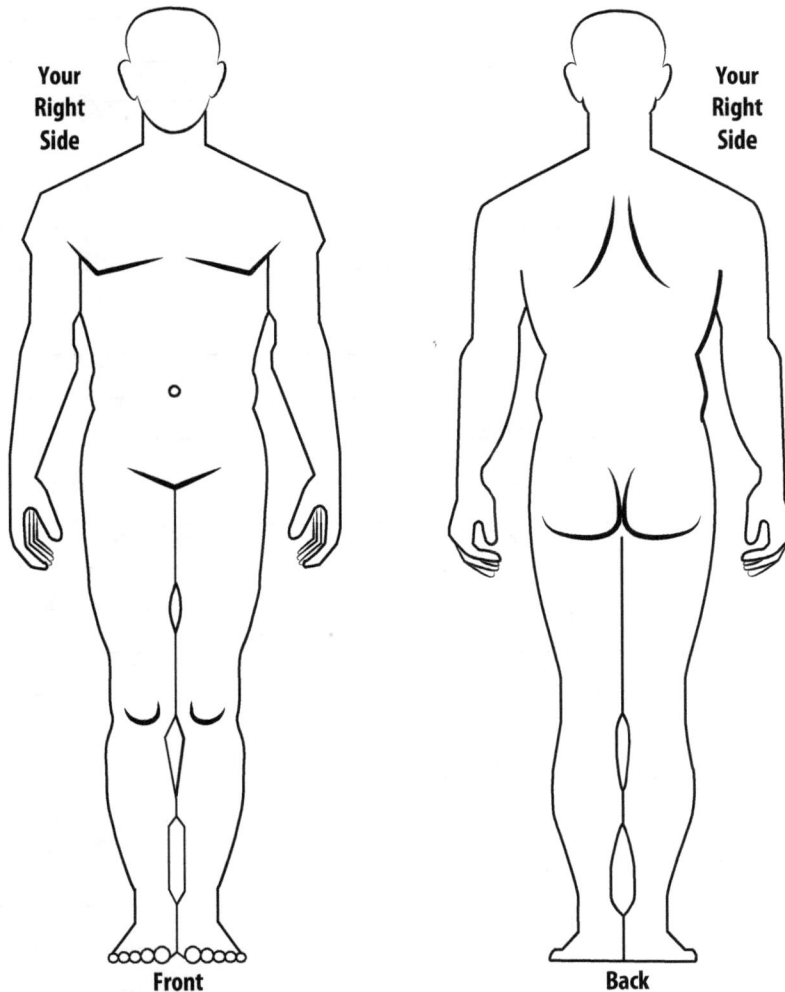

Your Right Side

Front

Your Right Side

Back

14

1 DAILY
TREATMENT PLAN

As you and your medical team develop new treatment plans, record your plan for the day including:
1.) New medications,
2.) Increases or decreases to medications,
3.) Exercises, physical therapy, or any other treatments,
4.) It will be especially helpful to record any side effects you experience as you add new treatments.
   This can help determine which types of treatments will work best for you.

Contact your care provider with any bad reactions or side effects to determine if you should discontinue the medication or treatment.

MEDICATION / TREATMENT	AMOUNT / TIME / COMMENTS

DAY_____ DATE_____ WEIGHT_____

INSTRUCTIONS:
1.) **Place an 'X'** on the chart below where the lines for the time of day and your level of pain meet.
2.) **Connect the points** on your DAILY PAIN CHART so your medical team can see when your status changed.
3.) **Refer to the EXAMPLES** in the front of this book for further direction.

2 DAILY PAIN CHART

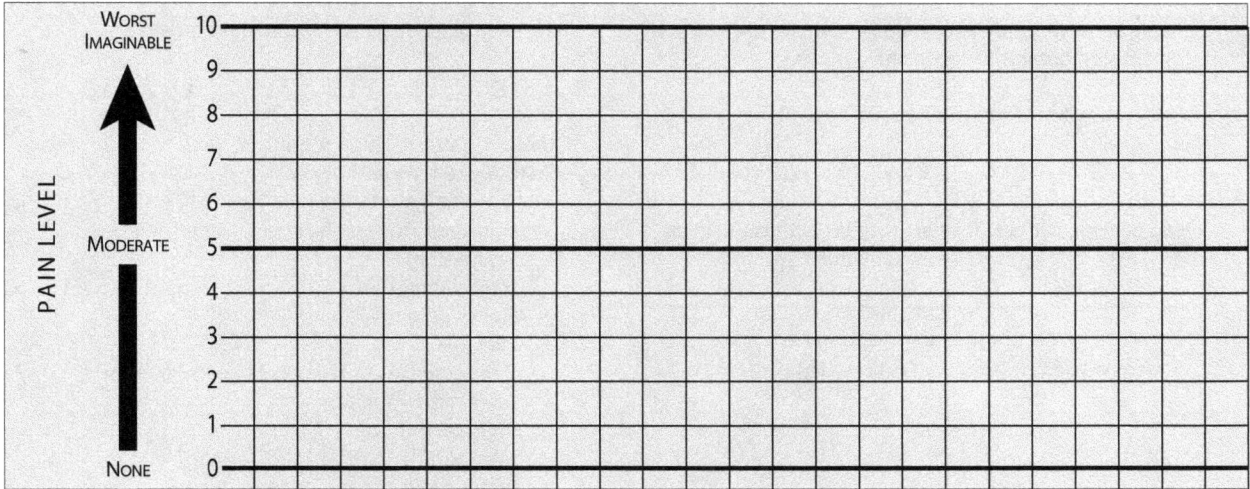

PAIN LEVEL

WORST IMAGINABLE — 10

9

8

7

6

MODERATE — 5

4

3

2

1

NONE — 0

3 DAILY MEDICATION

MEDICINE NAME / DOSE

6am 7 8 9 10 11 12pm 1 2 3 4 5 6pm 7 8 9 10 11 12am 1 2 3 4 5

1
2
3
4
5
6
7
8
9

4 DAILY PHYSIOLOGY

6am 7 8 9 10 11 12pm 1 2 3 4 5 6pm 7 8 9 10 11 12am 1 2 3 4 5

SLEEP

RESTROOM

NAUSEA / DIZZINESS

MEAL / SNACK

EXERCISE / PHYSICAL THERAPY

STRESS / ANXIETY

BLOOD PRESSURE

PULSE

5 DAILY
PAIN SUMMARY

Were there times during the day that you experienced unrelieved breakthrough pain? ____NO ____YES

How many times did this happen today?

1 2 3 4 5 6 7 8 9 10 more than 10

Did any specific activity start your breakthrough pain? ____NO ____YES: What activities?

_____

Put an "X" on the body diagram to show each place you've had *BREAKTHROUGH PAIN* today.

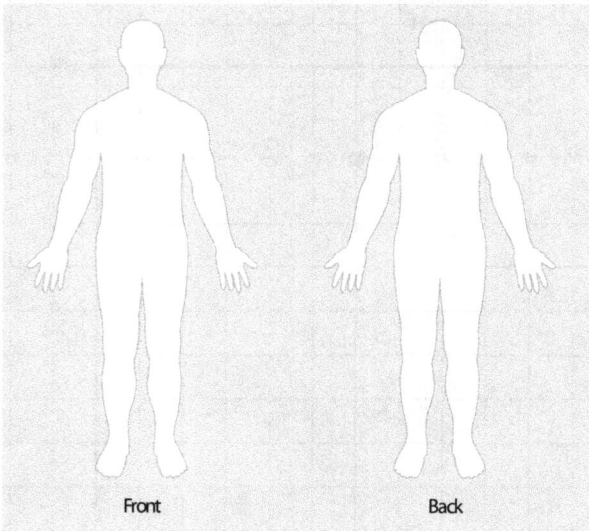

Front   Back

NON-DRUG THERAPIES
(other than prescription or other medicines)

_____

_____

ACTIVITIES/EXERCISE

_____

What was your average level of pain today?

0   1   2   3   4   5   6   7   8   9   10

Other than prescription medicine, did you do anything else today to relieve the pain? ____NO ____YES:
(Note any that you used.)
____ Non-prescription drugs (e.g., acetaminophen, ibuprofen)
____ Herbal remedies
____ Hot or cold packs
____ Exercise
____ Changing position (such as lying down or elevating your legs)
____ Physical therapy
____ Massage
____ Acupuncture
____ Rest
____ Prayer, meditation, guided imagery
____ Relaxation technique (hypnosis, biofeedback)
____ Creative technique (art or music therapy)
____ Other (e.g., specific chiropractic manipulation, osteopathic treatments):

_____

Check any of these common side effects that you've noticed after taking your pain medicine:
____ Drowsiness, sleepiness
____ Nausea, vomiting, upset stomach
____ Constipation
____ Lack of appetite
____ Other (describe):

_____

Did you sleep through the night? ____NO____YES

If not, how many times was your sleep disrupted? _____

How many hours did you sleep during the night? _____

COMMENTS AND MORE INFORMATION: Make notes for and about visits with your healthcare provider, side effects from treatments you may be experiencing, any problems you are having coping with your pain, and more about some of your previous answers or questions.

_____

_____

_____

6 DAILY BODY PAIN DIAGRAM

Mark each place on the diagram where you have had pain today by placing an 'X', circling the location, or shading the area .

Describe the type of pain:

Shooting	Deep
Tingling	Sharp
Numbness	Burning / Hot
Cold	Aching
Surface Pain	Gnawing / Biting
Stabbing	Electrical / Shocks
Dull	Other_____
Stinging	

COMMENTS AND MORE INFORMATION:

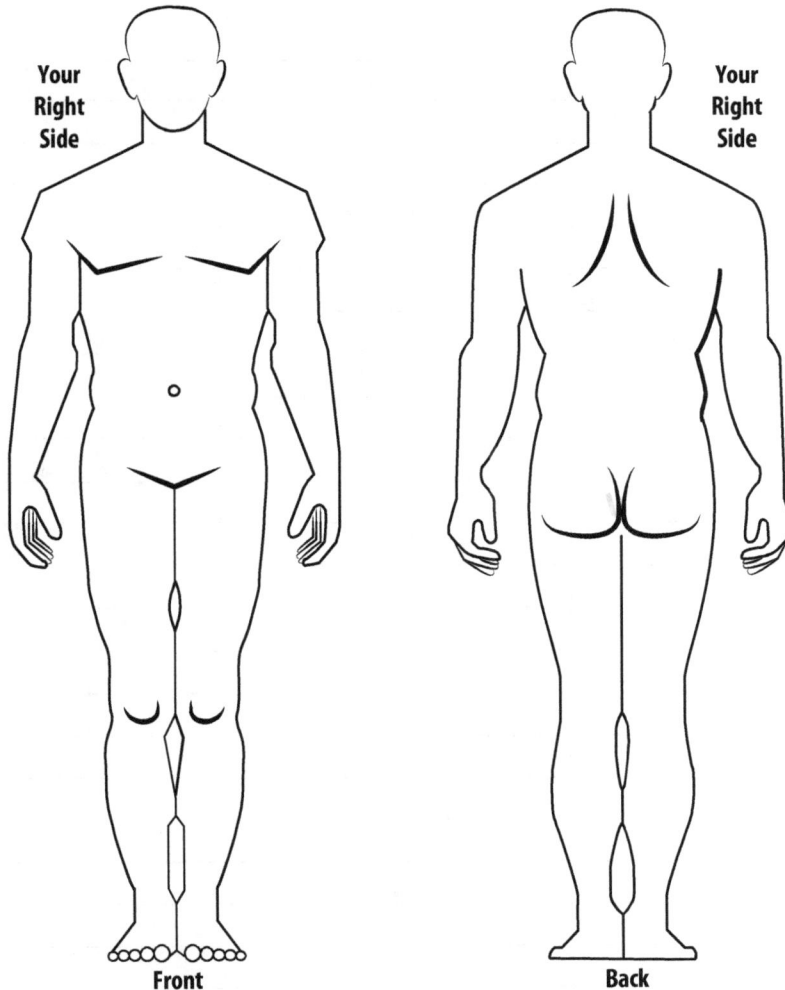

Your Right Side

Your Right Side

Front

Back

1 DAILY
TREATMENT PLAN

As you and your medical team develop new treatment plans, record your plan for the day including:
1.) New medications,
2.) Increases or decreases to medications,
3.) Exercises, physical therapy, or any other treatments,
4.) It will be especially helpful to record any side effects you experience as you add new treatments. This can help determine which types of treatments will work best for you.

Contact your care provider with any bad reactions or side effects to determine if you should discontinue the medication or treatment.

MEDICATION / TREATMENT	AMOUNT / TIME / COMMENTS

Day_____ Date_____ Weight_____

1.) **Place an 'X'** on the chart below where the lines for the time of day and your level of pain meet.
2.) **Connect the points** on your DAILY PAIN CHART so your medical team can see when your status changed.
3.) **Refer to the EXAMPLES** in the front of this book for further direction.

2 DAILY PAIN CHART

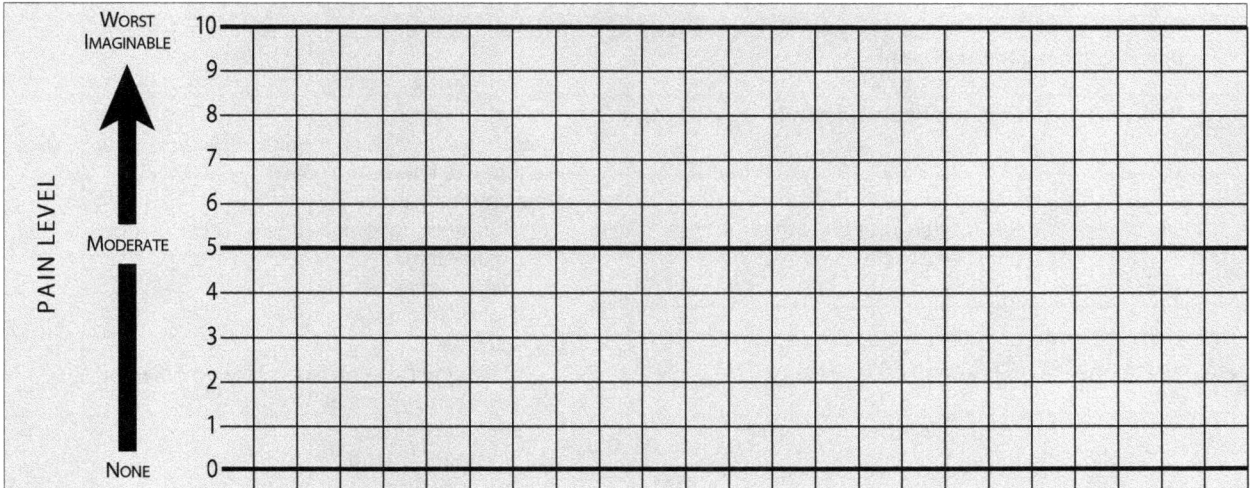

PAIN LEVEL

WORST IMAGINABLE — 10

9

8

7

6

MODERATE — 5

4

3

2

1

NONE — 0

3 DAILY MEDICATION

MEDICINE NAME / DOSE

	6am	7	8	9	10	11	12pm	1	2	3	4	5	6pm	7	8	9	10	11	12am	1	2	3	4	5
1																								
2																								
3																								
4																								
5																								
6																								
7																								
8																								
9																								

4 DAILY PHYSIOLOGY

	6am	7	8	9	10	11	12pm	1	2	3	4	5	6pm	7	8	9	10	11	12am	1	2	3	4	5
SLEEP																								
RESTROOM																								
NAUSEA / DIZZINESS																								
MEAL / SNACK																								
EXERCISE / PHYSICAL THERAPY																								
STRESS / ANXIETY																								
BLOOD PRESSURE																								
PULSE																								

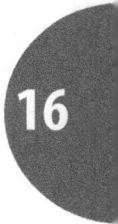

5 DAILY
PAIN SUMMARY

16

Were there times during the day that you experienced unrelieved breakthrough pain? ____NO ____YES

How many times did this happen today?

1   2   3   4   5   6   7   8   9   10   more than 10

Did any specific activity start your breakthrough pain?
____NO ____YES: What activities?

_____

Put an "X" on the body diagram to show each place you've had *BREAKTHROUGH PAIN* today.

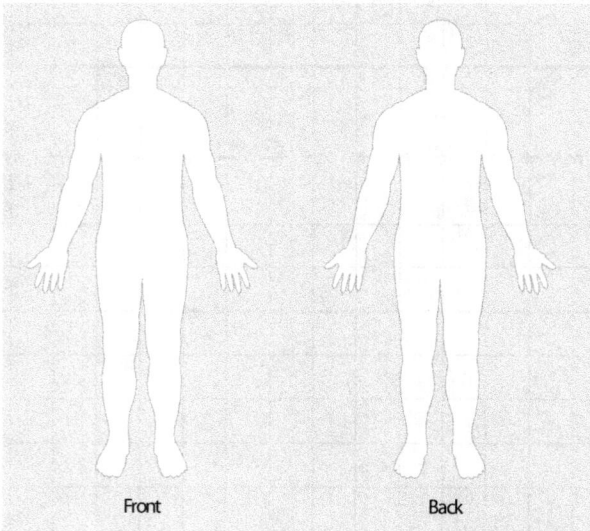

Front   Back

NON-DRUG THERAPIES
(other than prescription or other medicines)

_____

_____

ACTIVITIES/EXERCISE

_____

What was your average level of pain today?

0   1   2   3   4   5   6   7   8   9   10

Other than prescription medicine, did you do anything else today to relieve the pain? ____NO ____YES:
(Note any that you used.)
____ Non-prescription drugs (e.g., acetaminophen, ibuprofen)
____ Herbal remedies
____ Hot or cold packs
____ Exercise
____ Changing position (such as lying down or elevating your legs)
____ Physical therapy
____ Massage
____ Acupuncture
____ Rest
____ Prayer, meditation, guided imagery
____ Relaxation technique (hypnosis, biofeedback)
____ Creative technique (art or music therapy)
____ Other (e.g., specific chiropractic manipulation, osteopathic treatments):

_____

Check any of these common side effects that you've noticed after taking your pain medicine:
____ Drowsiness, sleepiness
____ Nausea, vomiting, upset stomach
____ Constipation
____ Lack of appetite
____ Other (describe):

_____

Did you sleep through the night? ____NO____YES

If not, how many times was your sleep disrupted? _____

How many hours did you sleep during the night? _____

COMMENTS AND MORE INFORMATION: Make notes for and about visits with your healthcare provider, side effects from treatments you may be experiencing, any problems you are having coping with your pain, and more about some of your previous answers or questions.

_____

_____

_____

6 DAILY BODY PAIN DIAGRAM

Mark each place on the diagram where you have had pain today by placing an 'X', circling the location, or shading the area .

Describe the type of pain:

Shooting	Deep
Tingling	Sharp
Numbness	Burning / Hot
Cold	Aching
Surface Pain	Gnawing / Biting
Stabbing	Electrical / Shocks
Dull	Other_____
Stinging	

COMMENTS AND MORE INFORMATION:

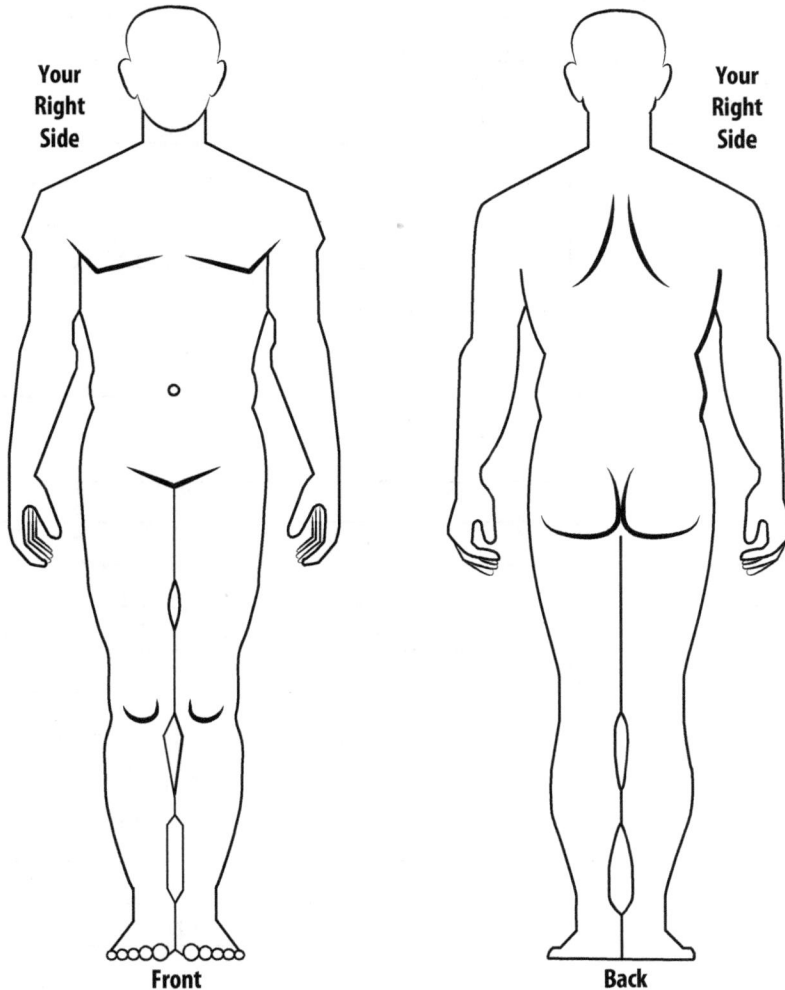

16

Your Right Side

Your Right Side

Front

Back

1 DAILY
TREATMENT PLAN

As you and your medical team develop new treatment plans, record your plan for the day including:
1.) New medications,
2.) Increases or decreases to medications,
3.) Exercises, physical therapy, or any other treatments,
4.) It will be especially helpful to record any side effects you experience as you add new treatments.
   This can help determine which types of treatments will work best for you.

Contact your care provider with any bad reactions or side effects to determine if you should discontinue
the medication or treatment.

MEDICATION / TREATMENT	AMOUNT / TIME / COMMENTS

17

INSTRUCTIONS:
1.) **Place an 'X'** on the chart below where the lines for the time of day and your level of pain meet.
2.) **Connect the points** on your DAILY PAIN CHART so your medical team can see when your status changed.
3.) **Refer to the EXAMPLES** in the front of this book for further direction.

DAY_____ DATE_____ WEIGHT_____

2 DAILY PAIN CHART

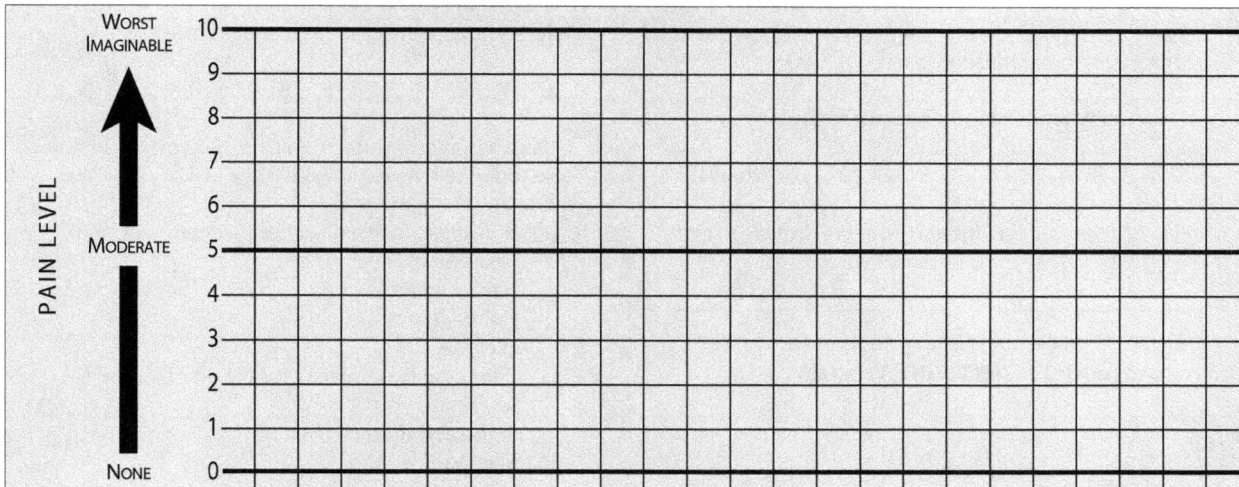

PAIN LEVEL

WORST IMAGINABLE — 10

9

8

7

6

MODERATE — 5

4

3

2

1

NONE — 0

17

3 DAILY MEDICATION

MEDICINE NAME / DOSE

6am 7 8 9 10 11 12pm 1 2 3 4 5 6pm 7 8 9 10 11 12am 1 2 3 4 5

1
2
3
4
5
6
7
8
9

4 DAILY PHYSIOLOGY

6am 7 8 9 10 11 12pm 1 2 3 4 5 6pm 7 8 9 10 11 12am 1 2 3 4 5

SLEEP
RESTROOM
NAUSEA / DIZZINESS
MEAL / SNACK
EXERCISE / PHYSICAL THERAPY
STRESS / ANXIETY
BLOOD PRESSURE
PULSE

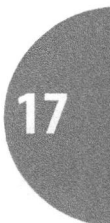

5 DAILY
PAIN SUMMARY

Were there times during the day that you experienced unrelieved breakthrough pain? ____NO ____YES

How many times did this happen today?

1   2   3   4   5   6   7   8   9   10   more than 10

Did any specific activity start your breakthrough pain? ____NO ____YES: What activities?

_____

Put an "X" on the body diagram to show each place you've had **BREAKTHROUGH PAIN** today.

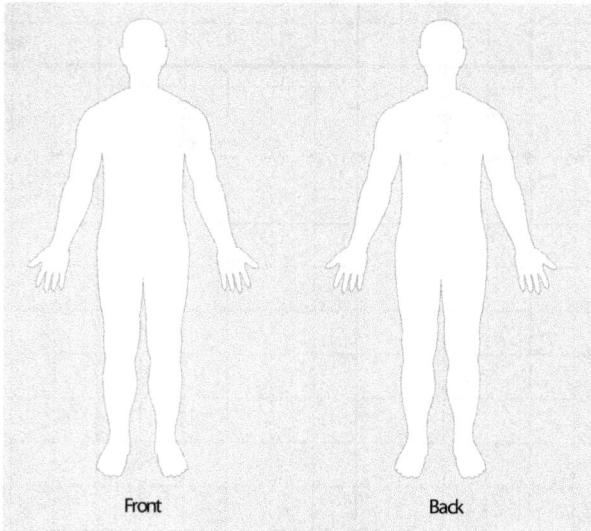

Front   Back

NON-DRUG THERAPIES
(other than prescription or other medicines)

_____

_____

ACTIVITIES/EXERCISE

_____

_____

What was your average level of pain today?

0   1   2   3   4   5   6   7   8   9   10

Other than prescription medicine, did you do anything else today to relieve the pain? ____NO ____YES: (Note any that you used.)
____ Non-prescription drugs (e.g., acetaminophen, ibuprofen)
____ Herbal remedies
____ Hot or cold packs
____ Exercise
____ Changing position (such as lying down or elevating your legs)
____ Physical therapy
____ Massage
____ Acupuncture
____ Rest
____ Prayer, meditation, guided imagery
____ Relaxation technique (hypnosis, biofeedback)
____ Creative technique (art or music therapy)
____ Other (e.g., specific chiropractic manipulation, osteopathic treatments):

_____

Check any of these common side effects that you've noticed after taking your pain medicine:
____ Drowsiness, sleepiness
____ Nausea, vomiting, upset stomach
____ Constipation
____ Lack of appetite
____ Other (describe):

_____

Did you sleep through the night? ____NO____YES

If not, how many times was your sleep disrupted? _____

How many hours did you sleep during the night? _____

COMMENTS AND MORE INFORMATION: Make notes for and about visits with your healthcare provider, side effects from treatments you may be experiencing, any problems you are having coping with your pain, and more about some of your previous answers or questions.

_____

_____

_____

6 DAILY BODY PAIN DIAGRAM

Mark each place on the diagram where you have had pain today by placing an 'X', circling the location, or shading the area .

Describe the type of pain:

Shooting   Deep
Tingling   Sharp
Numbness   Burning / Hot
Cold   Aching
Surface Pain   Gnawing / Biting
Stabbing   Electrical / Shocks
Dull   Other_____
Stinging

COMMENTS AND MORE INFORMATION:

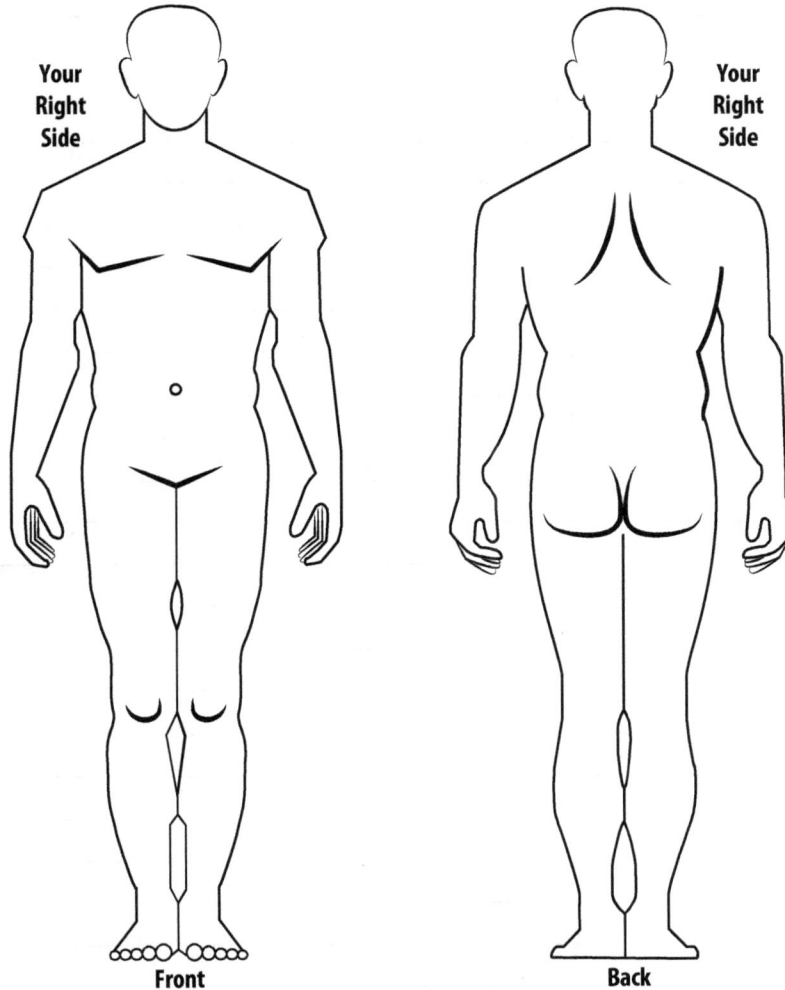

17

Your
Right
Side

Your
Right
Side

Front

Back

1 DAILY
TREATMENT PLAN

As you and your medical team develop new treatment plans, record your plan for the day including:
1.) New medications,
2.) Increases or decreases to medications,
3.) Exercises, physical therapy, or any other treatments,
4.) It will be especially helpful to record any side effects you experience as you add new treatments.
   This can help determine which types of treatments will work best for you.

Contact your care provider with any bad reactions or side effects to determine if you should discontinue the medication or treatment.

MEDICATION / TREATMENT	AMOUNT / TIME / COMMENTS

18

DAY_____ DATE_____ WEIGHT_____

INSTRUCTIONS:
1.) **Place an 'X'** on the chart below where the lines for the time of day and your level of pain meet.
2.) **Connect the points** on your DAILY PAIN CHART so your medical team can see when your status changed.
3.) **Refer to the EXAMPLES** in the front of this book for further direction.

2 DAILY PAIN CHART

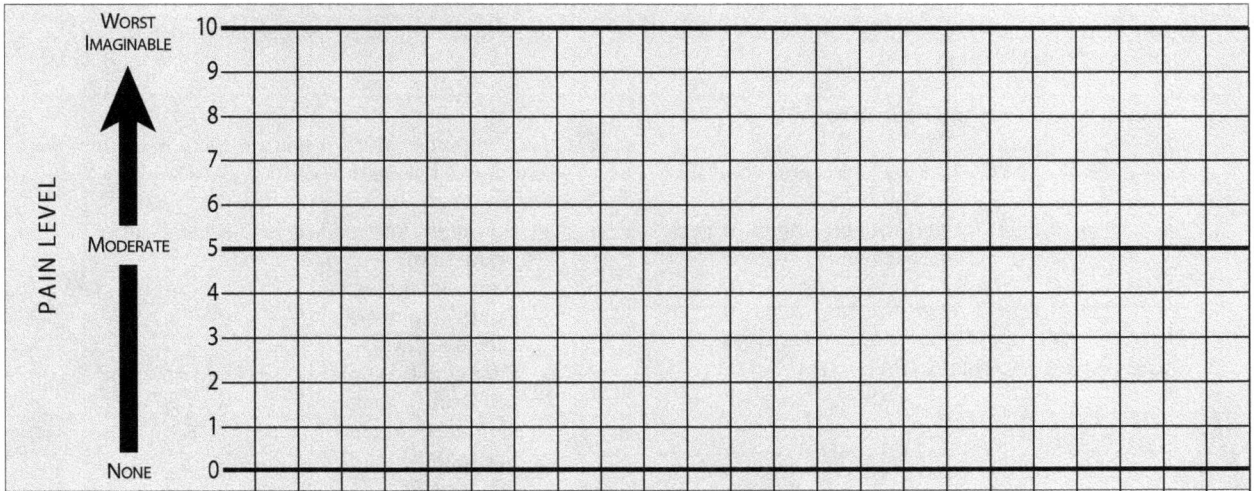

WORST IMAGINABLE — 10

PAIN LEVEL

MODERATE — 5

NONE — 0

9 8 7 6 4 3 2 1

3 DAILY MEDICATION

MEDICINE NAME / DOSE

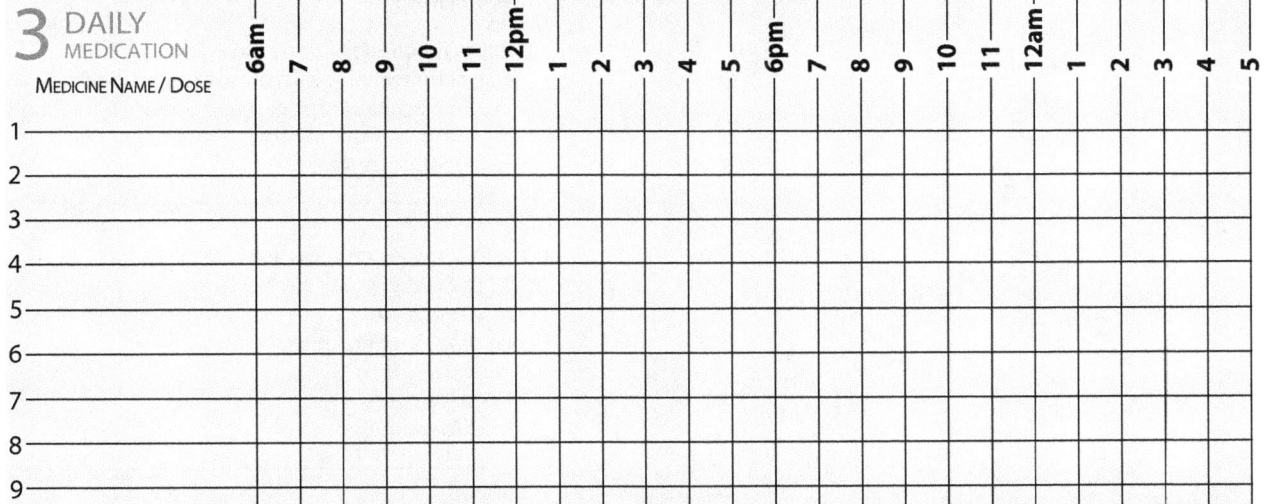

6am 7 8 9 10 11 12pm 1 2 3 4 5 6pm 7 8 9 10 11 12am 1 2 3 4 5

1
2
3
4
5
6
7
8
9

18

4 DAILY PHYSIOLOGY

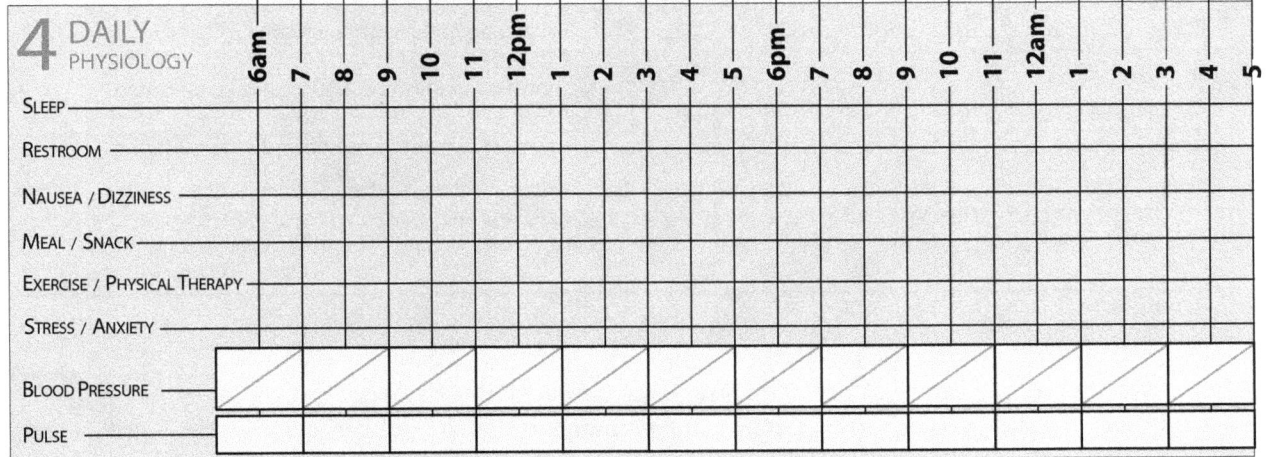

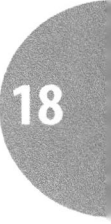

6am 7 8 9 10 11 12pm 1 2 3 4 5 6pm 7 8 9 10 11 12am 1 2 3 4 5

SLEEP

RESTROOM

NAUSEA / DIZZINESS

MEAL / SNACK

EXERCISE / PHYSICAL THERAPY

STRESS / ANXIETY

BLOOD PRESSURE

PULSE

5 DAILY
PAIN SUMMARY

Were there times during the day that you experienced unrelieved breakthrough pain? ____NO ____YES

How many times did this happen today?

1 2 3 4 5 6 7 8 9 10 more than 10

Did any specific activity start your breakthrough pain? ____NO ____YES: What activities?

_____

Put an "X" on the body diagram to show each place you've had **BREAKTHROUGH PAIN** today.

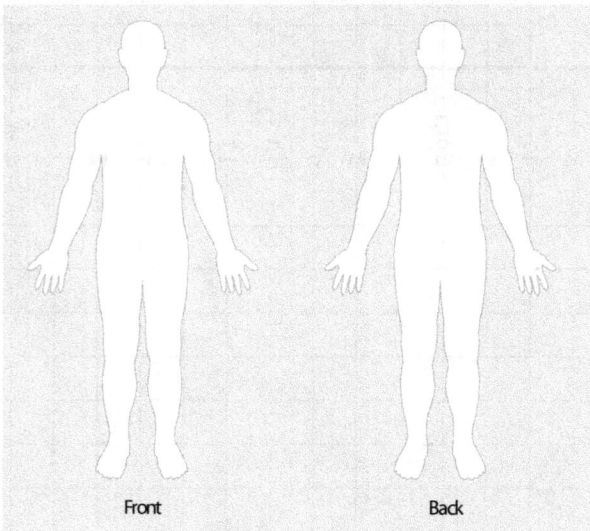

Front   Back

NON-DRUG THERAPIES
(other than prescription or other medicines)

_____
_____

ACTIVITIES/EXERCISE

_____

What was your average level of pain today?

0 1 2 3 4 5 6 7 8 9 10

Other than prescription medicine, did you do anything else today to relieve the pain? ____NO ____YES: (Note any that you used.)
____ Non-prescription drugs (e.g., acetaminophen, ibuprofen)
____ Herbal remedies
____ Hot or cold packs
____ Exercise
____ Changing position (such as lying down or elevating your legs)
____ Physical therapy
____ Massage
____ Acupuncture
____ Rest
____ Prayer, meditation, guided imagery
____ Relaxation technique (hypnosis, biofeedback)
____ Creative technique (art or music therapy)
____ Other (e.g., specific chiropractic manipulation, osteopathic treatments):

_____

Check any of these common side effects that you've noticed after taking your pain medicine:
____ Drowsiness, sleepiness
____ Nausea, vomiting, upset stomach
____ Constipation
____ Lack of appetite
____ Other (describe):

_____

Did you sleep through the night? ____NO____YES

If not, how many times was your sleep disrupted? _____

How many hours did you sleep during the night? _____

COMMENTS AND MORE INFORMATION: Make notes for and about visits with your healthcare provider, side effects from treatments you may be experiencing, any problems you are having coping with your pain, and more about some of your previous answers or questions.

_____
_____
_____

18

6 DAILY BODY PAIN DIAGRAM

Mark each place on the diagram where you have had pain today by placing an 'X', circling the location, or shading the area .

Describe the type of pain:

Shooting	Deep
Tingling	Sharp
Numbness	Burning / Hot
Cold	Aching
Surface Pain	Gnawing / Biting
Stabbing	Electrical / Shocks
Dull	Other_____
Stinging	

COMMENTS AND MORE INFORMATION:

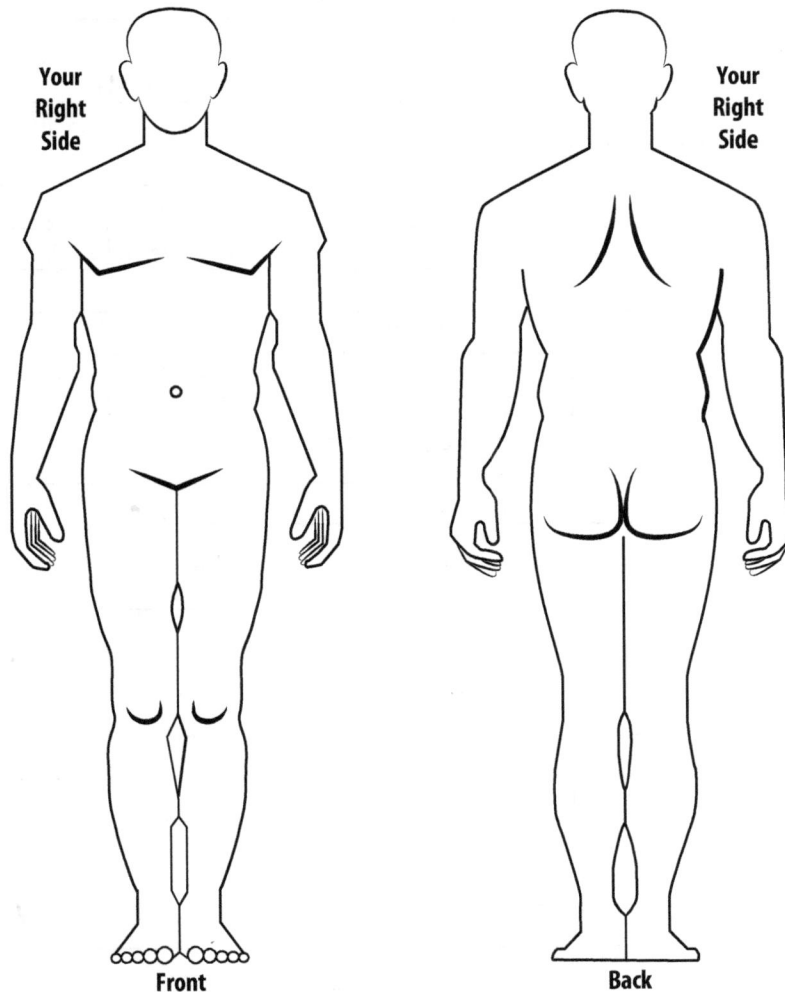

Your Right Side

Your Right Side

18

Front

Back

1 DAILY
TREATMENT PLAN

As you and your medical team develop new treatment plans, record your plan for the day including:
1.) New medications,
2.) Increases or decreases to medications,
3.) Exercises, physical therapy, or any other treatments,
4.) It will be especially helpful to record any side effects you experience as you add new treatments.
   This can help determine which types of treatments will work best for you.

Contact your care provider with any bad reactions or side effects to determine if you should discontinue the medication or treatment.

MEDICATION / TREATMENT	AMOUNT / TIME / COMMENTS

19

DAY_____ DATE_____ WEIGHT_____

INSTRUCTIONS:
1.) **Place an 'X'** on the chart below where the lines for the time of day and your level of pain meet.
2.) **Connect the points** on your DAILY PAIN CHART so your medical team can see when your status changed.
3.) **Refer to the EXAMPLES** in the front of this book for further direction.

2 DAILY PAIN CHART

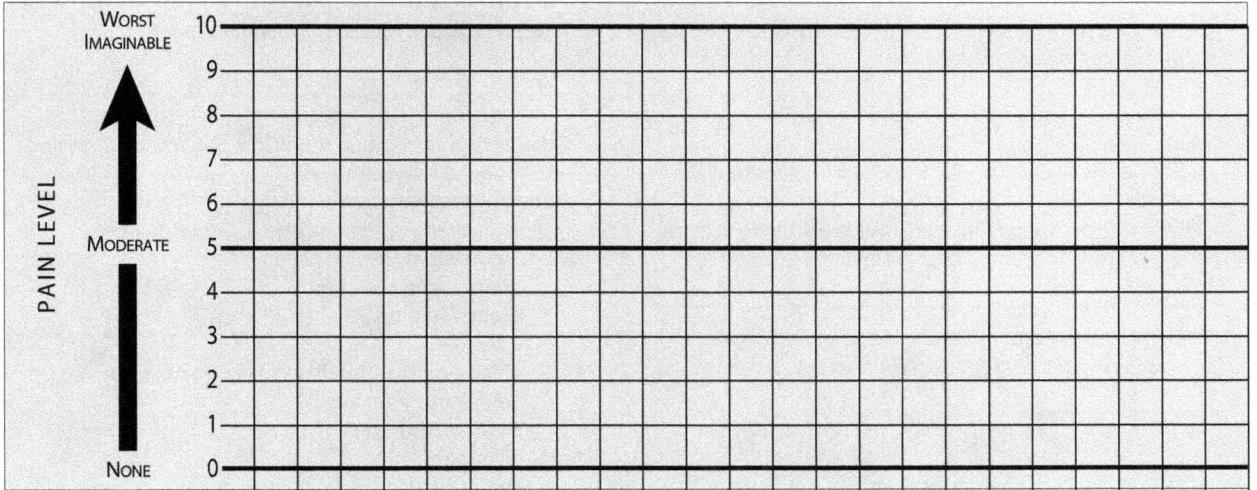

PAIN LEVEL

WORST IMAGINABLE — 10
9
8
7
6
MODERATE — 5
4
3
2
1
NONE — 0

3 DAILY MEDICATION

MEDICINE NAME / DOSE

Times: 6am, 7, 8, 9, 10, 11, 12pm, 1, 2, 3, 4, 5, 6pm, 7, 8, 9, 10, 11, 12am, 1, 2, 3, 4, 5

1
2
3
4
5
6
7
8
9

4 DAILY PHYSIOLOGY

Times: 6am, 7, 8, 9, 10, 11, 12pm, 1, 2, 3, 4, 5, 6pm, 7, 8, 9, 10, 11, 12am, 1, 2, 3, 4, 5

SLEEP
RESTROOM
NAUSEA / DIZZINESS
MEAL / SNACK
EXERCISE / PHYSICAL THERAPY
STRESS / ANXIETY
BLOOD PRESSURE
PULSE

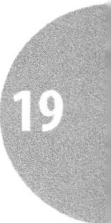
19

5 DAILY
PAIN SUMMARY

Were there times during the day that you experienced unrelieved breakthrough pain? ____NO ____YES

How many times did this happen today?

1 2 3 4 5 6 7 8 9 10 more than 10

Did any specific activity start your breakthrough pain? ____NO ____YES: What activities?

_____

Put an "X" on the body diagram to show each place you've had **BREAKTHROUGH PAIN** today.

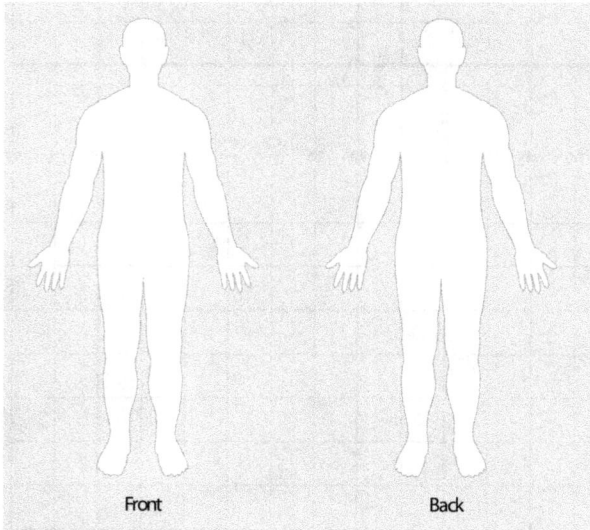

Front   Back

NON-DRUG THERAPIES
(other than prescription or other medicines)

_____

_____

ACTIVITIES/EXERCISE

_____

What was your average level of pain today?

0 1 2 3 4 5 6 7 8 9 10

Other than prescription medicine, did you do anything else today to relieve the pain? ____NO ____YES: (Note any that you used.)
____ Non-prescription drugs (e.g., acetaminophen, ibuprofen)
____ Herbal remedies
____ Hot or cold packs
____ Exercise
____ Changing position (such as lying down or elevating your legs)
____ Physical therapy
____ Massage
____ Acupuncture
____ Rest
____ Prayer, meditation, guided imagery
____ Relaxation technique (hypnosis, biofeedback)
____ Creative technique (art or music therapy)
____ Other (e.g., specific chiropractic manipulation, osteopathic treatments):

_____

Check any of these common side effects that you've noticed after taking your pain medicine:
____ Drowsiness, sleepiness
____ Nausea, vomiting, upset stomach
____ Constipation
____ Lack of appetite
____ Other (describe):

_____

Did you sleep through the night? ____NO____YES

If not, how many times was your sleep disrupted? _____

How many hours did you sleep during the night? _____

COMMENTS AND MORE INFORMATION: Make notes for and about visits with your healthcare provider, side effects from treatments you may be experiencing, any problems you are having coping with your pain, and more about some of your previous answers or questions.

_____

_____

19

6 DAILY BODY PAIN DIAGRAM

Mark each place on the diagram where you have had pain today by placing an 'X', circling the location, or shading the area .

Describe the type of pain:

Shooting	Deep
Tingling	Sharp
Numbness	Burning / Hot
Cold	Aching
Surface Pain	Gnawing / Biting
Stabbing	Electrical / Shocks
Dull	Other_____
Stinging	

COMMENTS AND MORE INFORMATION:

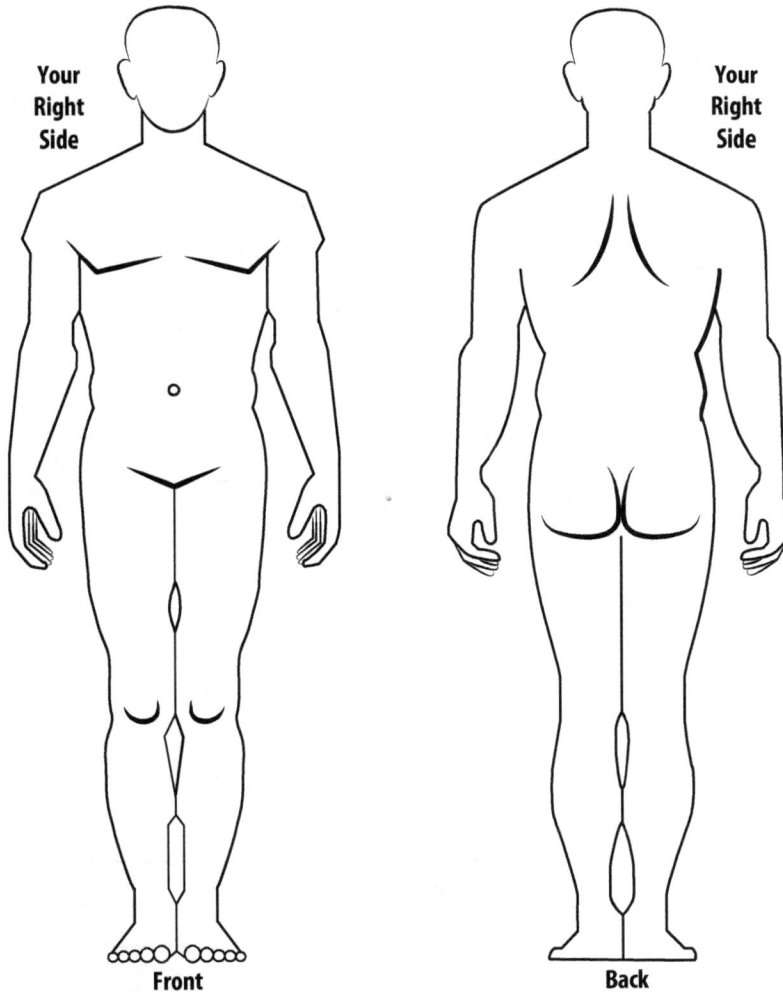

Your Right Side

Your Right Side

Front

Back

19

1 DAILY
TREATMENT PLAN

As you and your medical team develop new treatment plans, record your plan for the day including:
1.) New medications,
2.) Increases or decreases to medications,
3.) Exercises, physical therapy, or any other treatments,
4.) It will be especially helpful to record any side effects you experience as you add new treatments.
   This can help determine which types of treatments will work best for you.

Contact your care provider with any bad reactions or side effects to determine if you should discontinue the medication or treatment.

MEDICATION / TREATMENT	AMOUNT / TIME / COMMENTS

20

DAY_____ DATE_____ WEIGHT_____

INSTRUCTIONS:
1.) **Place an 'X'** on the chart below where the lines for the time of day and your level of pain meet.
2.) **Connect the points** on your DAILY PAIN CHART so your medical team can see when your status changed.
3.) **Refer to the EXAMPLES** in the front of this book for further direction.

2 DAILY PAIN CHART

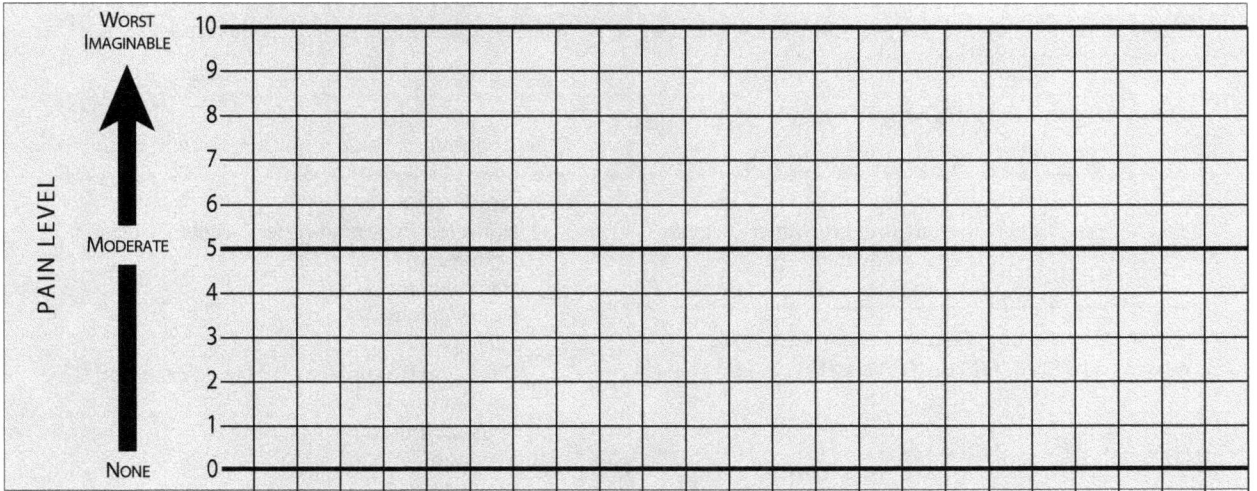

3 DAILY MEDICATION

MEDICINE NAME / DOSE

	6am	7	8	9	10	11	12pm	1	2	3	4	5	6pm	7	8	9	10	11	12am	1	2	3	4	5
1																								
2																								
3																								
4																								
5																								
6																								
7																								
8																								
9																								

4 DAILY PHYSIOLOGY

	6am	7	8	9	10	11	12pm	1	2	3	4	5	6pm	7	8	9	10	11	12am	1	2	3	4	5
SLEEP																								
RESTROOM																								
NAUSEA / DIZZINESS																								
MEAL / SNACK																								
EXERCISE / PHYSICAL THERAPY																								
STRESS / ANXIETY																								
BLOOD PRESSURE																								
PULSE																								

5 DAILY
PAIN SUMMARY

Were there times during the day that you experienced unrelieved breakthrough pain? ____NO ____YES

How many times did this happen today?

1 2 3 4 5 6 7 8 9 10 more than 10

Did any specific activity start your breakthrough pain? ____NO ____YES: What activities?

_____

Put an "X" on the body diagram to show each place you've had **BREAKTHROUGH PAIN** today.

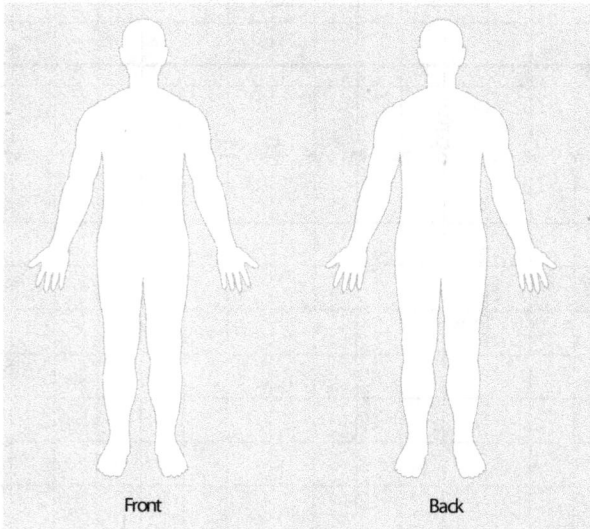

Front   Back

NON-DRUG THERAPIES
(other than prescription or other medicines)

_____

_____

ACTIVITIES/EXERCISE

_____

What was your average level of pain today?

0   1   2   3   4   5   6   7   8   9   10

Other than prescription medicine, did you do anything else today to relieve the pain? ____NO ____YES: (Note any that you used.)
____ Non-prescription drugs (e.g., acetaminophen, ibuprofen)
____ Herbal remedies
____ Hot or cold packs
____ Exercise
____ Changing position (such as lying down or elevating your legs)
____ Physical therapy
____ Massage
____ Acupuncture
____ Rest
____ Prayer, meditation, guided imagery
____ Relaxation technique (hypnosis, biofeedback)
____ Creative technique (art or music therapy)
____ Other (e.g., specific chiropractic manipulation, osteopathic treatments):

_____

Check any of these common side effects that you've noticed after taking your pain medicine:
____ Drowsiness, sleepiness
____ Nausea, vomiting, upset stomach
____ Constipation
____ Lack of appetite
____ Other (describe):

_____

Did you sleep through the night? ____NO____YES

If not, how many times was your sleep disrupted? _____

How many hours did you sleep during the night? _____

COMMENTS AND MORE INFORMATION: Make notes for and about visits with your healthcare provider, side effects from treatments you may be experiencing, any problems you are having coping with your pain, and more about some of your previous answers or questions.

_____

_____

_____

20

6 DAILY BODY PAIN DIAGRAM

Mark each place on the diagram where you have had pain today by placing an 'X', circling the location, or shading the area .

Describe the type of pain:

Shooting	Deep
Tingling	Sharp
Numbness	Burning / Hot
Cold	Aching
Surface Pain	Gnawing / Biting
Stabbing	Electrical / Shocks
Dull	Other_____
Stinging	

COMMENTS AND MORE INFORMATION:

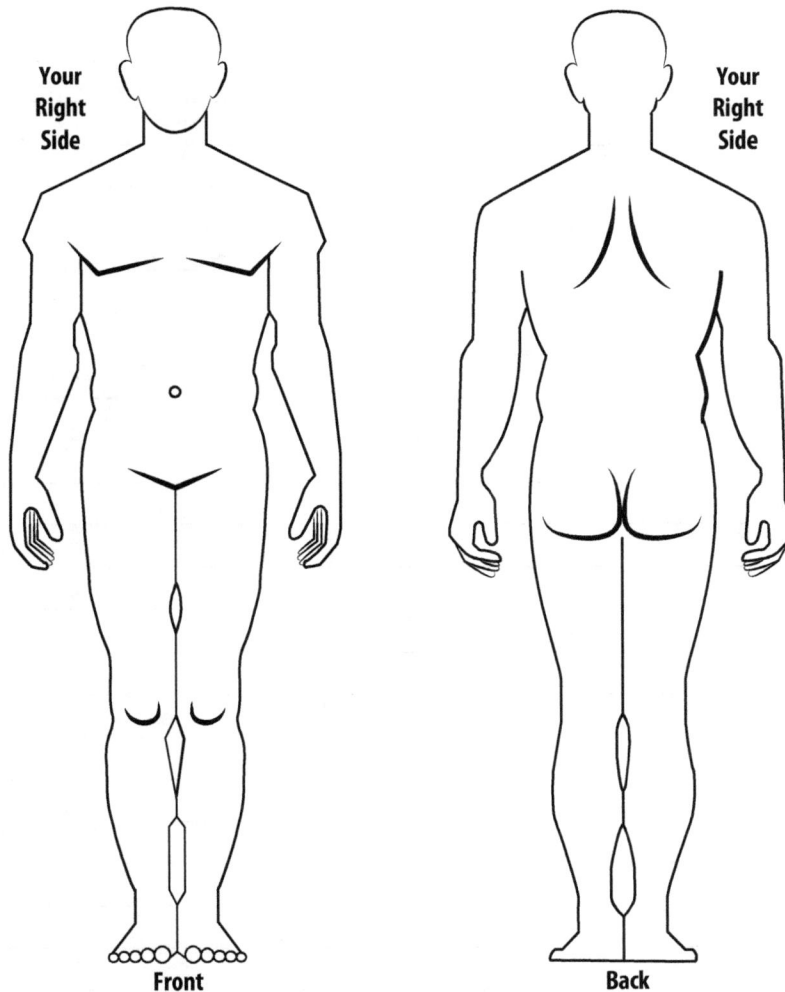

Your Right Side

Your Right Side

Front

Back

20

1 DAILY
TREATMENT PLAN

As you and your medical team develop new treatment plans, record your plan for the day including:
1.) New medications,
2.) Increases or decreases to medications,
3.) Exercises, physical therapy, or any other treatments,
4.) It will be especially helpful to record any side effects you experience as you add new treatments.
   This can help determine which types of treatments will work best for you.

Contact your care provider with any bad reactions or side effects to determine if you should discontinue the medication or treatment.

MEDICATION / TREATMENT	AMOUNT / TIME / COMMENTS

21

DAY_____ DATE_____ WEIGHT_____

INSTRUCTIONS:
1.) **Place an 'X'** on the chart below where the lines for the time of day and your level of pain meet.
2.) **Connect the points** on your DAILY PAIN CHART so your medical team can see when your status changed.
3.) **Refer to the EXAMPLES** in the front of this book for further direction.

2 DAILY PAIN CHART

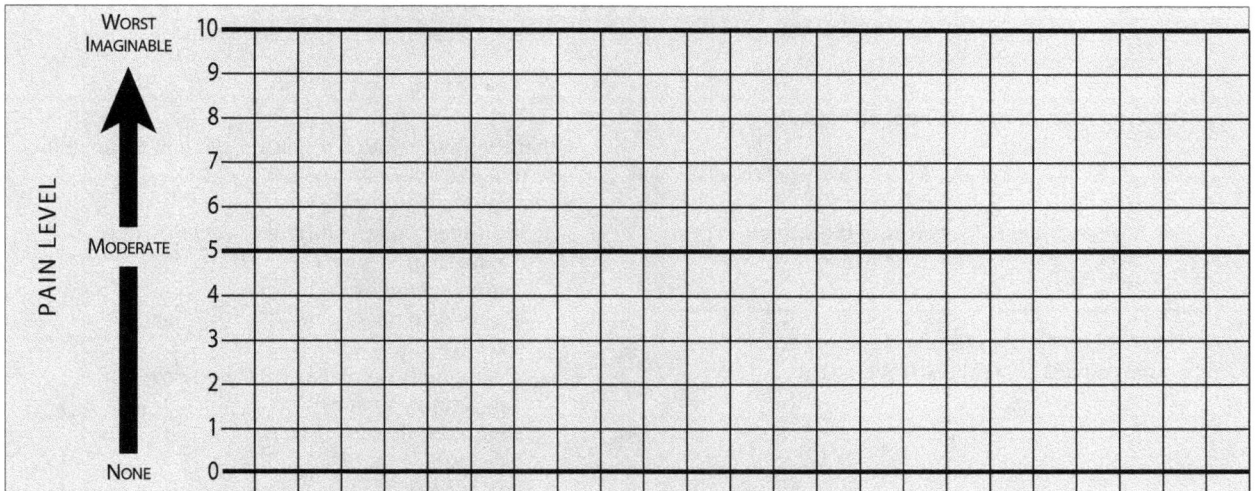

PAIN LEVEL

WORST IMAGINABLE — 10
9
8
7
6
MODERATE — 5
4
3
2
1
NONE — 0

3 DAILY MEDICATION

MEDICINE NAME / DOSE

	6am	7	8	9	10	11	12pm	1	2	3	4	5	6pm	7	8	9	10	11	12am	1	2	3	4	5
1																								
2																								
3																								
4																								
5																								
6																								
7																								
8																								
9																								

4 DAILY PHYSIOLOGY

	6am	7	8	9	10	11	12pm	1	2	3	4	5	6pm	7	8	9	10	11	12am	1	2	3	4	5
SLEEP																								
RESTROOM																								
NAUSEA / DIZZINESS																								
MEAL / SNACK																								
EXERCISE / PHYSICAL THERAPY																								
STRESS / ANXIETY																								
BLOOD PRESSURE																								
PULSE																								

21

5 DAILY
PAIN SUMMARY

Were there times during the day that you experienced unrelieved breakthrough pain? _____NO _____YES

How many times did this happen today?

1   2   3   4   5   6   7   8   9   10   more than 10

Did any specific activity start your breakthrough pain? _____NO _____YES: What activities?

_____

Put an "X" on the body diagram to show each place you've had **BREAKTHROUGH PAIN** today.

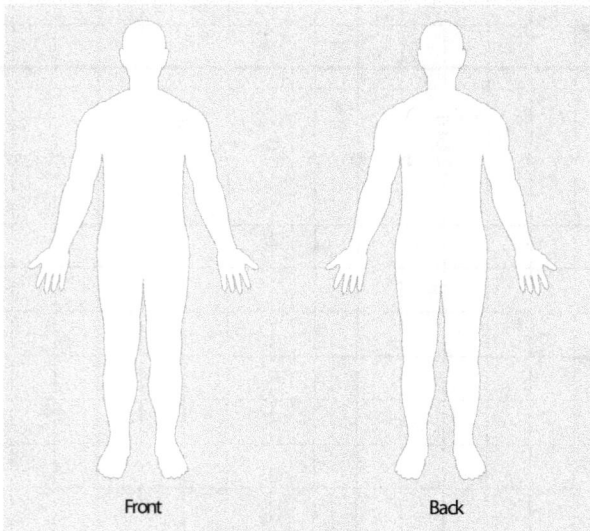

Front   Back

NON-DRUG THERAPIES
(other than prescription or other medicines)

_____

_____

ACTIVITIES/EXERCISE

_____

_____

What was your average level of pain today?

0   1   2   3   4   5   6   7   8   9   10

Other than prescription medicine, did you do anything else today to relieve the pain? _____NO _____YES: (Note any that you used.)

_____ Non-prescription drugs (e.g., acetaminophen, ibuprofen)
_____ Herbal remedies
_____ Hot or cold packs
_____ Exercise
_____ Changing position (such as lying down or elevating your legs)
_____ Physical therapy
_____ Massage
_____ Acupuncture
_____ Rest
_____ Prayer, meditation, guided imagery
_____ Relaxation technique (hypnosis, biofeedback)
_____ Creative technique (art or music therapy)
_____ Other (e.g., specific chiropractic manipulation, osteopathic treatments):

_____

Check any of these common side effects that you've noticed after taking your pain medicine:
_____ Drowsiness, sleepiness
_____ Nausea, vomiting, upset stomach
_____ Constipation
_____ Lack of appetite
_____ Other (describe):

_____

Did you sleep through the night? _____NO_____YES

If not, how many times was your sleep disrupted? _____

How many hours did you sleep during the night? _____

COMMENTS AND MORE INFORMATION: Make notes for and about visits with your healthcare provider, side effects from treatments you may be experiencing, any problems you are having coping with your pain, and more about some of your previous answers or questions.

_____

_____

_____

21

6 DAILY BODY PAIN DIAGRAM

Mark each place on the diagram where you have had pain today by placing an 'X', circling the location, or shading the area .

Describe the type of pain:

Shooting	Deep
Tingling	Sharp
Numbness	Burning / Hot
Cold	Aching
Surface Pain	Gnawing / Biting
Stabbing	Electrical / Shocks
Dull	Other_____
Stinging	

COMMENTS AND MORE INFORMATION:

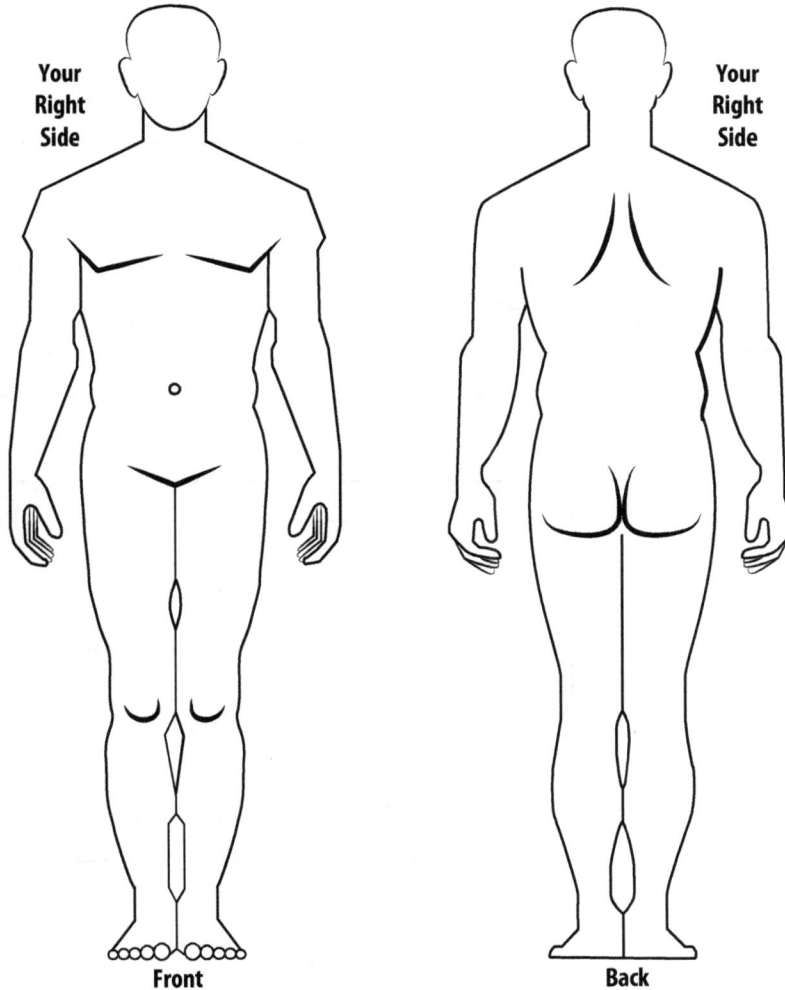

Your Right Side

Your Right Side

Front

Back

21

22

1 DAILY
TREATMENT PLAN

As you and your medical team develop new treatment plans, record your plan for the day including:
1.) New medications,
2.) Increases or decreases to medications,
3.) Exercises, physical therapy, or any other treatments,
4.) It will be especially helpful to record any side effects you experience as you add new treatments.
     This can help determine which types of treatments will work best for you.

Contact your care provider with any bad reactions or side effects to determine if you should discontinue
the medication or treatment.

MEDICATION / TREATMENT	AMOUNT / TIME / COMMENTS

INSTRUCTIONS:
1.) **Place an 'X'** on the chart below where the lines for the time of day and your level of pain meet.
2.) **Connect the points** on your DAILY PAIN CHART so your medical team can see when your status changed.
3.) **Refer to the EXAMPLES** in the front of this book for further direction.

DAY_____ DATE_____ WEIGHT_____

22

2 DAILY PAIN CHART

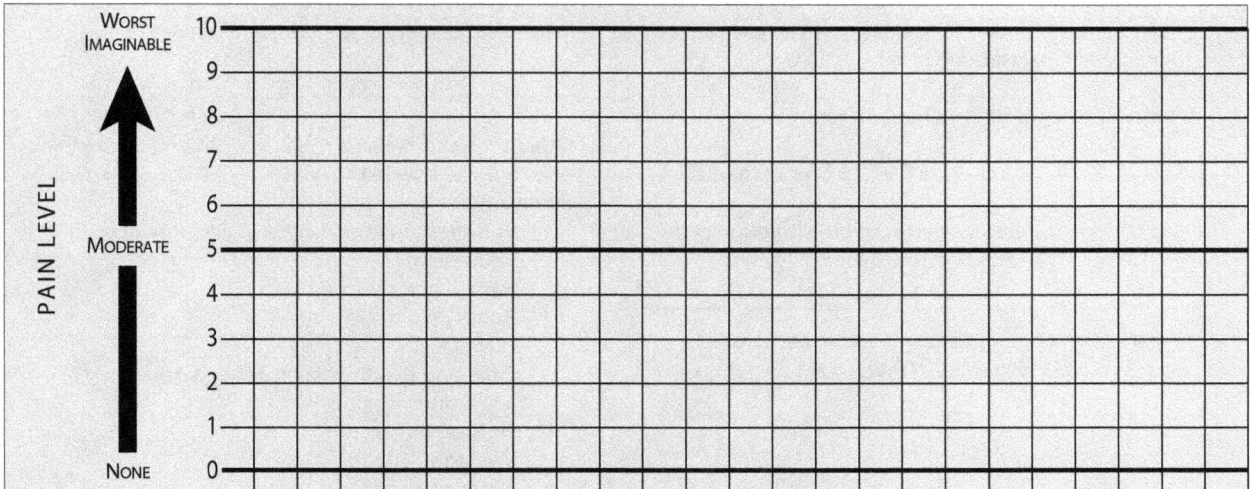

PAIN LEVEL

WORST IMAGINABLE — 10
9
8
7
6
MODERATE — 5
4
3
2
1
NONE — 0

Time axis: 6am, 7, 8, 9, 10, 11, 12pm, 1, 2, 3, 4, 5, 6pm, 7, 8, 9, 10, 11, 12am, 1, 2, 3, 4, 5

3 DAILY MEDICATION

MEDICINE NAME / DOSE

1
2
3
4
5
6
7
8
9

4 DAILY PHYSIOLOGY

SLEEP
RESTROOM
NAUSEA / DIZZINESS
MEAL / SNACK
EXERCISE / PHYSICAL THERAPY
STRESS / ANXIETY
BLOOD PRESSURE
PULSE

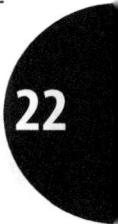

5 DAILY
PAIN SUMMARY

Were there times during the day that you experienced unrelieved breakthrough pain? ____NO ____YES

How many times did this happen today?

1 2 3 4 5 6 7 8 9 10 more than 10

Did any specific activity start your breakthrough pain? ____NO ____YES: What activities?

_____

Put an "X" on the body diagram to show each place you've had **BREAKTHROUGH PAIN** today.

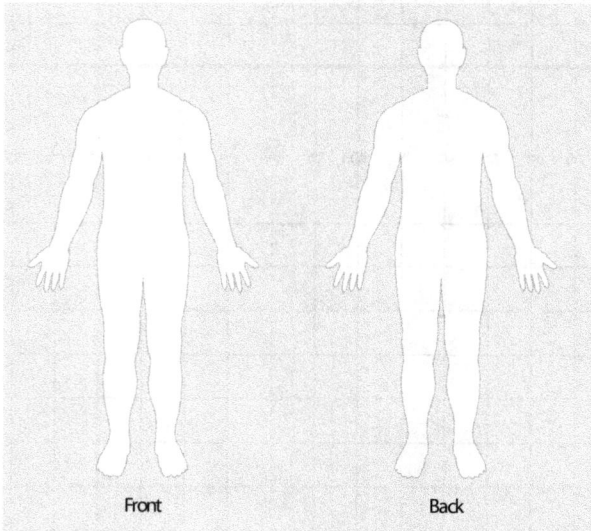

Front   Back

NON-DRUG THERAPIES
(other than prescription or other medicines)

_____
_____

ACTIVITIES/EXERCISE

_____
_____

What was your average level of pain today?

0 1 2 3 4 5 6 7 8 9 10

Other than prescription medicine, did you do anything else today to relieve the pain? ____NO ____YES: (Note any that you used.)
____ Non-prescription drugs (e.g., acetaminophen, ibuprofen)
____ Herbal remedies
____ Hot or cold packs
____ Exercise
____ Changing position (such as lying down or elevating your legs)
____ Physical therapy
____ Massage
____ Acupuncture
____ Rest
____ Prayer, meditation, guided imagery
____ Relaxation technique (hypnosis, biofeedback)
____ Creative technique (art or music therapy)
____ Other (e.g., specific chiropractic manipulation, osteopathic treatments):

_____

Check any of these common side effects that you've noticed after taking your pain medicine:
____ Drowsiness, sleepiness
____ Nausea, vomiting, upset stomach
____ Constipation
____ Lack of appetite
____ Other (describe):

_____

Did you sleep through the night? ____NO____YES

If not, how many times was your sleep disrupted? _____

How many hours did you sleep during the night? _____

COMMENTS AND MORE INFORMATION: Make notes for and about visits with your healthcare provider, side effects from treatments you may be experiencing, any problems you are having coping with your pain, and more about some of your previous answers or questions.

_____
_____
_____

6 DAILY BODY PAIN DIAGRAM

Mark each place on the diagram where you have had pain today by placing an 'X', circling the location, or shading the area .

Describe the type of pain:

Shooting	Deep
Tingling	Sharp
Numbness	Burning / Hot
Cold	Aching
Surface Pain	Gnawing / Biting
Stabbing	Electrical / Shocks
Dull	Other_____
Stinging	

COMMENTS AND MORE INFORMATION:

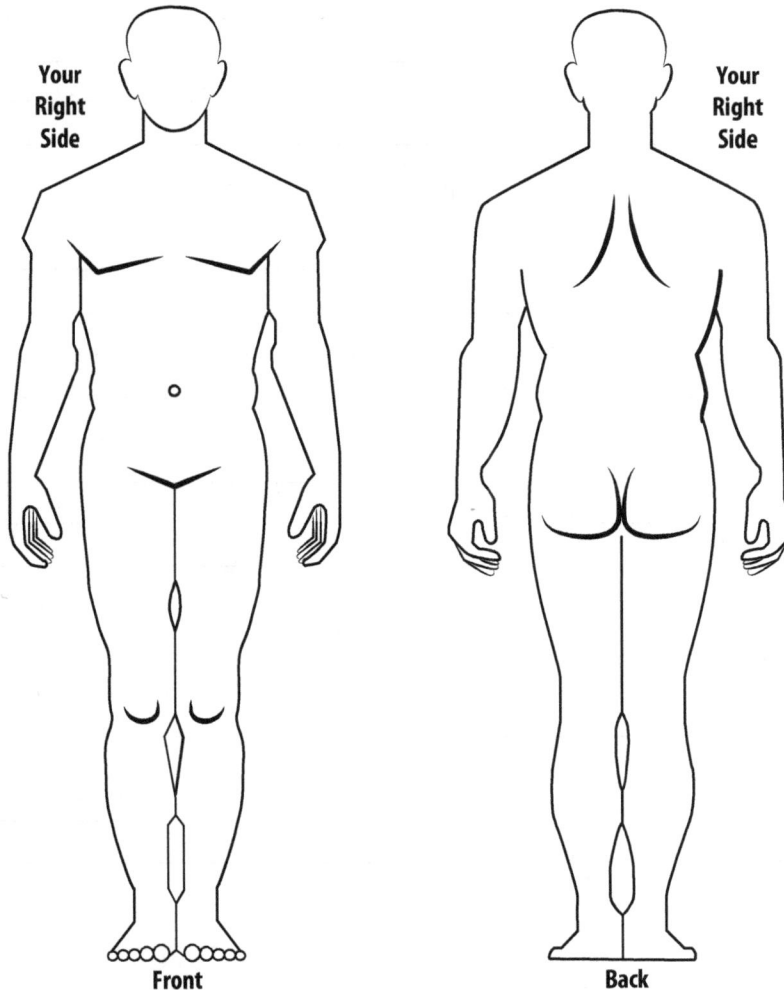

Your Right Side

Your Right Side

Front

Back

1 DAILY
TREATMENT PLAN

As you and your medical team develop new treatment plans, record your plan for the day including:
1.) New medications,
2.) Increases or decreases to medications,
3.) Exercises, physical therapy, or any other treatments,
4.) It will be especially helpful to record any side effects you experience as you add new treatments.
    This can help determine which types of treatments will work best for you.

Contact your care provider with any bad reactions or side effects to determine if you should discontinue the medication or treatment.

23

MEDICATION / TREATMENT	AMOUNT / TIME / COMMENTS

INSTRUCTIONS:

DAY_____ DATE_____ WEIGHT_____

1.) **Place an 'X'** on the chart below where the lines for the time of day and your level of pain meet.
2.) **Connect the points** on your DAILY PAIN CHART so your medical team can see when your status changed.
3.) **Refer to the EXAMPLES** in the front of this book for further direction.

2 DAILY PAIN CHART

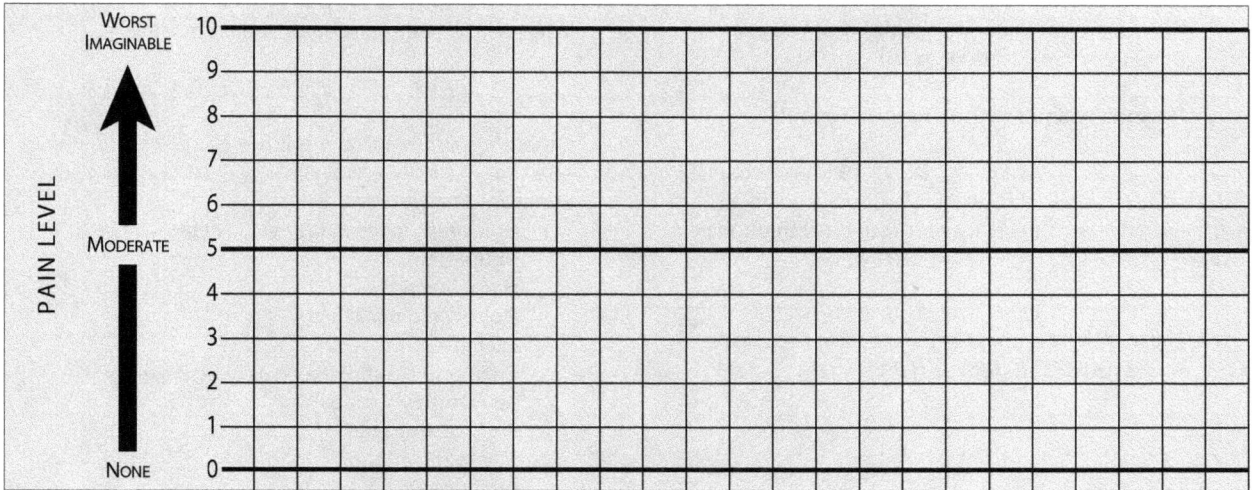

PAIN LEVEL

WORST IMAGINABLE — 10

9

8

7

6

MODERATE — 5

4

3

2

1

NONE — 0

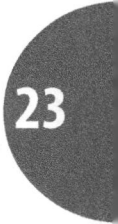

23

3 DAILY MEDICATION

MEDICINE NAME / DOSE

Times: 6am, 7, 8, 9, 10, 11, 12pm, 1, 2, 3, 4, 5, 6pm, 7, 8, 9, 10, 11, 12am, 1, 2, 3, 4, 5

1
2
3
4
5
6
7
8
9

4 DAILY PHYSIOLOGY

Times: 6am, 7, 8, 9, 10, 11, 12pm, 1, 2, 3, 4, 5, 6pm, 7, 8, 9, 10, 11, 12am, 1, 2, 3, 4, 5

SLEEP

RESTROOM

NAUSEA / DIZZINESS

MEAL / SNACK

EXERCISE / PHYSICAL THERAPY

STRESS / ANXIETY

BLOOD PRESSURE

PULSE

5 DAILY
PAIN SUMMARY

23

Were there times during the day that you experienced unrelieved breakthrough pain? ____NO ____YES

How many times did this happen today?

1   2   3   4   5   6   7   8   9   10   more than 10

Did any specific activity start your breakthrough pain? ____NO ____YES: What activities?

_____

Put an "X" on the body diagram to show each place you've had *BREAKTHROUGH PAIN* today.

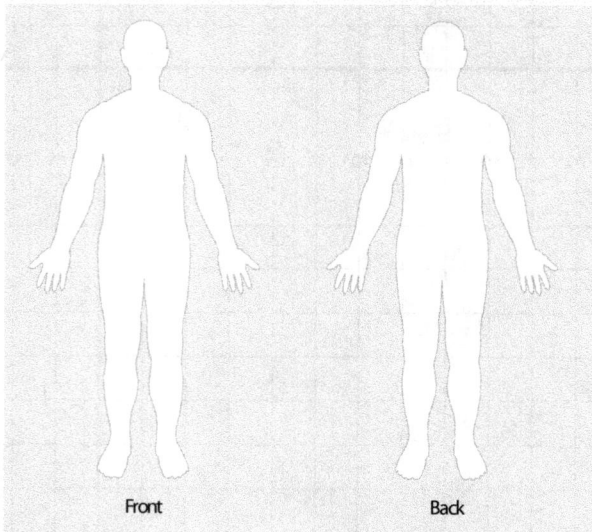

Front   Back

NON-DRUG THERAPIES
(other than prescription or other medicines)

_____

_____

ACTIVITIES/EXERCISE

_____

What was your average level of pain today?

0   1   2   3   4   5   6   7   8   9   10

Other than prescription medicine, did you do anything else today to relieve the pain? ____NO ____YES:
(Note any that you used.)
____ Non-prescription drugs (e.g., acetaminophen, ibuprofen)
____ Herbal remedies
____ Hot or cold packs
____ Exercise
____ Changing position (such as lying down or elevating your legs)
____ Physical therapy
____ Massage
____ Acupuncture
____ Rest
____ Prayer, meditation, guided imagery
____ Relaxation technique (hypnosis, biofeedback)
____ Creative technique (art or music therapy)
____ Other (e.g., specific chiropractic manipulation, osteopathic treatments):

_____

Check any of these common side effects that you've noticed after taking your pain medicine:
____ Drowsiness, sleepiness
____ Nausea, vomiting, upset stomach
____ Constipation
____ Lack of appetite
____ Other (describe):

_____

Did you sleep through the night? ____NO____YES

If not, how many times was your sleep disrupted? _____

How many hours did you sleep during the night? _____

COMMENTS AND MORE INFORMATION: Make notes for and about visits with your healthcare provider, side effects from treatments you may be experiencing, any problems you are having coping with your pain, and more about some of your previous answers or questions.

_____

_____

6 DAILY BODY PAIN DIAGRAM

Mark each place on the diagram where you have had pain today by placing an 'X', circling the location, or shading the area .

Describe the type of pain:

Shooting   Deep
Tingling   Sharp
Numbness   Burning / Hot
Cold   Aching
Surface Pain   Gnawing / Biting
Stabbing   Electrical / Shocks
Dull   Other_____
Stinging

COMMENTS AND MORE INFORMATION:

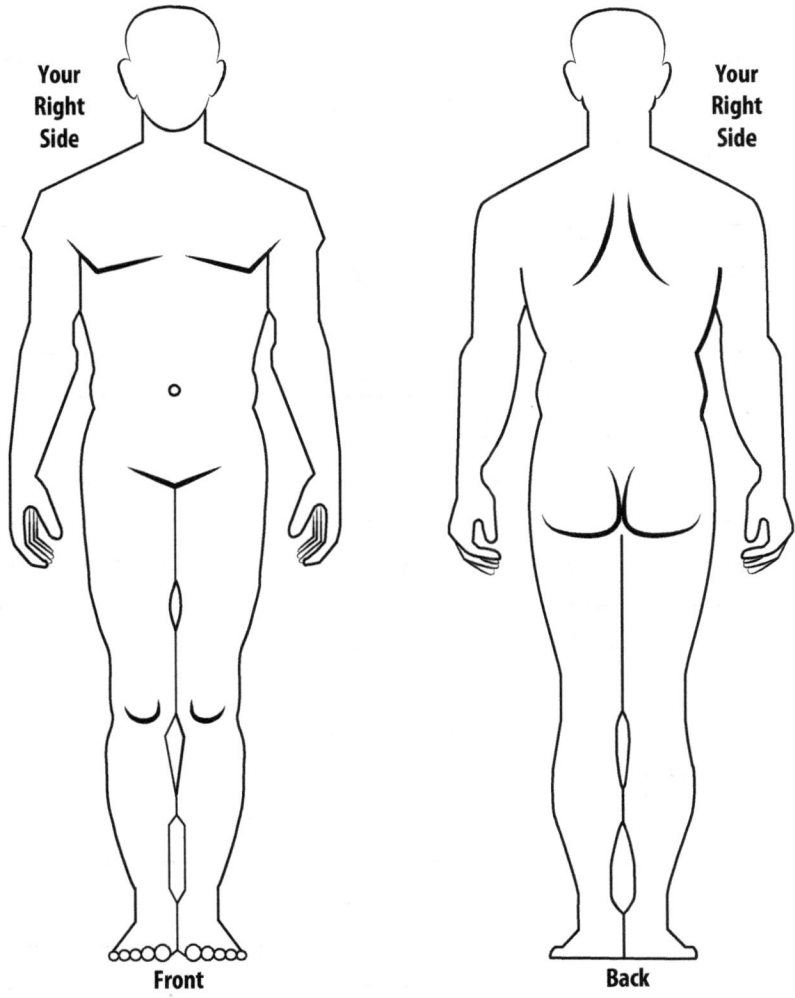

23

Your Right Side

Your Right Side

Front

Back

1 DAILY
TREATMENT PLAN

As you and your medical team develop new treatment plans, record your plan for the day including:
1.) New medications,
2.) Increases or decreases to medications,
3.) Exercises, physical therapy, or any other treatments,
4.) It will be especially helpful to record any side effects you experience as you add new treatments.
This can help determine which types of treatments will work best for you.

Contact your care provider with any bad reactions or side effects to determine if you should discontinue the medication or treatment.

24

MEDICATION / TREATMENT	AMOUNT / TIME / COMMENTS

INSTRUCTIONS:

Day_____ Date_____ Weight_____

1.) **Place an 'X'** on the chart below where the lines for the time of day and your level of pain meet.
2.) **Connect the points** on your DAILY PAIN CHART so your medical team can see when your status changed.
3.) **Refer to the EXAMPLES** in the front of this book for further direction.

2 DAILY PAIN CHART

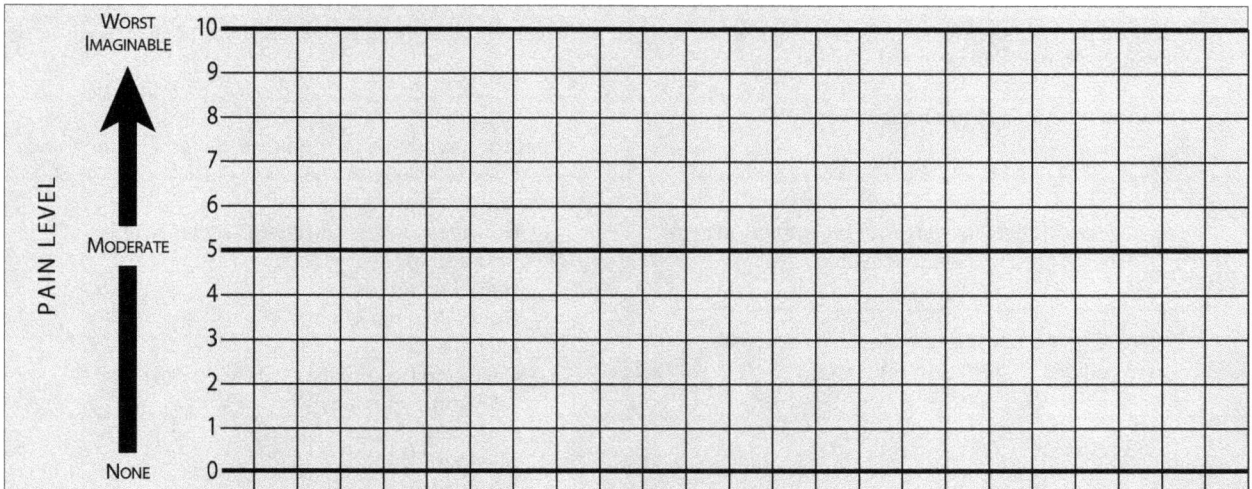

PAIN LEVEL

WORST IMAGINABLE — 10
9
8
7
6
MODERATE — 5
4
3
2
1
NONE — 0

3 DAILY MEDICATION

MEDICINE NAME / DOSE

6am 7 8 9 10 11 12pm 1 2 3 4 5 6pm 7 8 9 10 11 12am 1 2 3 4 5

1
2
3
4
5
6
7
8
9

4 DAILY PHYSIOLOGY

6am 7 8 9 10 11 12pm 1 2 3 4 5 6pm 7 8 9 10 11 12am 1 2 3 4 5

SLEEP
RESTROOM
NAUSEA / DIZZINESS
MEAL / SNACK
EXERCISE / PHYSICAL THERAPY
STRESS / ANXIETY
BLOOD PRESSURE
PULSE

24

5 DAILY
PAIN SUMMARY

Were there times during the day that you experienced unrelieved breakthrough pain? ____NO ____YES

How many times did this happen today?

1 2 3 4 5 6 7 8 9 10 more than 10

Did any specific activity start your breakthrough pain? ____NO ____YES: What activities?

_____

Put an "X" on the body diagram to show each place you've had **BREAKTHROUGH PAIN** today.

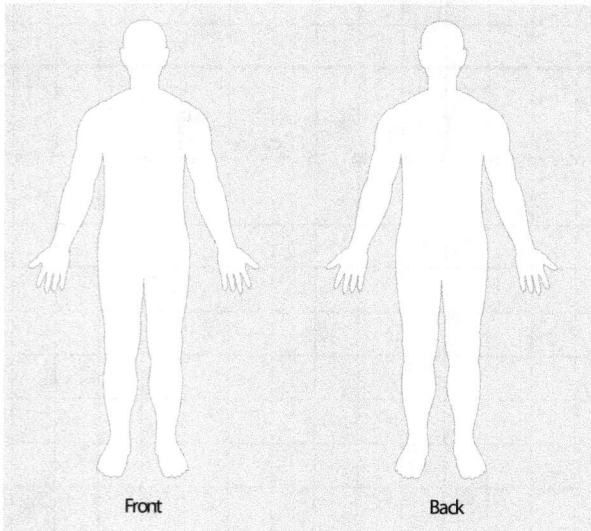

Front   Back

NON-DRUG THERAPIES
(other than prescription or other medicines)

_____

_____

ACTIVITIES/EXERCISE

_____

_____

What was your average level of pain today?

0 1 2 3 4 5 6 7 8 9 10

Other than prescription medicine, did you do anything else today to relieve the pain? ____NO ____YES: (Note any that you used.)
____ Non-prescription drugs (e.g., acetaminophen, ibuprofen)
____ Herbal remedies
____ Hot or cold packs
____ Exercise
____ Changing position (such as lying down or elevating your legs)
____ Physical therapy
____ Massage
____ Acupuncture
____ Rest
____ Prayer, meditation, guided imagery
____ Relaxation technique (hypnosis, biofeedback)
____ Creative technique (art or music therapy)
____ Other (e.g., specific chiropractic manipulation, osteopathic treatments):

_____

Check any of these common side effects that you've noticed after taking your pain medicine:
____ Drowsiness, sleepiness
____ Nausea, vomiting, upset stomach
____ Constipation
____ Lack of appetite
____ Other (describe):

_____

Did you sleep through the night? ____NO____YES

If not, how many times was your sleep disrupted? _____

How many hours did you sleep during the night? _____

COMMENTS AND MORE INFORMATION: Make notes for and about visits with your healthcare provider, side effects from treatments you may be experiencing, any problems you are having coping with your pain, and more about some of your previous answers or questions.

_____

_____

_____

6 DAILY BODY PAIN DIAGRAM

Mark each place on the diagram where you have had pain today by placing an 'X', circling the location, or shading the area .

Describe the type of pain:

Shooting	Deep
Tingling	Sharp
Numbness	Burning / Hot
Cold	Aching
Surface Pain	Gnawing / Biting
Stabbing	Electrical / Shocks
Dull	Other_____
Stinging	

COMMENTS AND MORE INFORMATION:

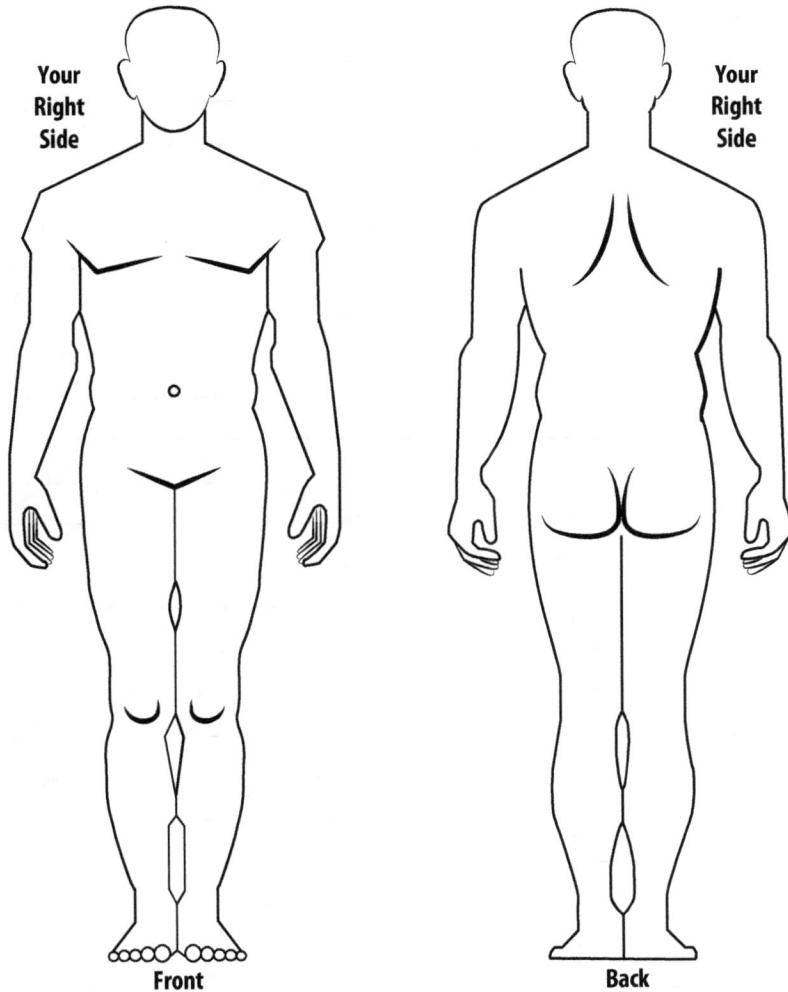

24

Your
Right
Side

Your
Right
Side

Front

Back

1 DAILY
TREATMENT PLAN

As you and your medical team develop new treatment plans, record your plan for the day including:
1.) New medications,
2.) Increases or decreases to medications,
3.) Exercises, physical therapy, or any other treatments,
4.) It will be especially helpful to record any side effects you experience as you add new treatments.
    This can help determine which types of treatments will work best for you.

Contact your care provider with any bad reactions or side effects to determine if you should discontinue
the medication or treatment.

Medication / Treatment	Amount / Time / Comments

25

DAY_____ DATE_____ WEIGHT_____

INSTRUCTIONS:
1.) **Place an 'X'** on the chart below where the lines for the time of day and your level of pain meet.
2.) **Connect the points** on your DAILY PAIN CHART so your medical team can see when your status changed.
3.) **Refer to the EXAMPLES** in the front of this book for further direction.

2 DAILY PAIN CHART

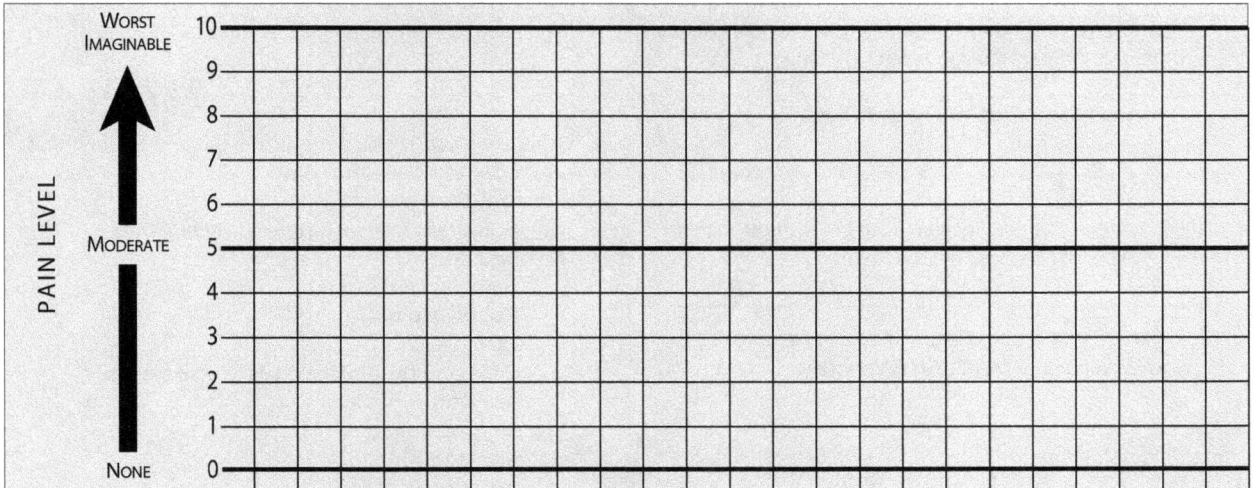

PAIN LEVEL

WORST IMAGINABLE	10
	9
	8
	7
	6
MODERATE	5
	4
	3
	2
	1
NONE	0

3 DAILY MEDICATION

MEDICINE NAME / DOSE

6am 7 8 9 10 11 12pm 1 2 3 4 5 6pm 7 8 9 10 11 12am 1 2 3 4 5

1
2
3
4
5
6
7
8
9

25

4 DAILY PHYSIOLOGY

6am 7 8 9 10 11 12pm 1 2 3 4 5 6pm 7 8 9 10 11 12am 1 2 3 4 5

SLEEP
RESTROOM
NAUSEA / DIZZINESS
MEAL / SNACK
EXERCISE / PHYSICAL THERAPY
STRESS / ANXIETY
BLOOD PRESSURE
PULSE

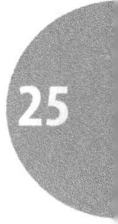

5 DAILY
PAIN SUMMARY

Were there times during the day that you experienced unrelieved breakthrough pain? ____NO ____YES

How many times did this happen today?

1   2   3   4   5   6   7   8   9   10   more than 10

Did any specific activity start your breakthrough pain?
____NO   ____YES: What activities?

_____

Put an "X" on the body diagram to show each place you've had **BREAKTHROUGH PAIN** today.

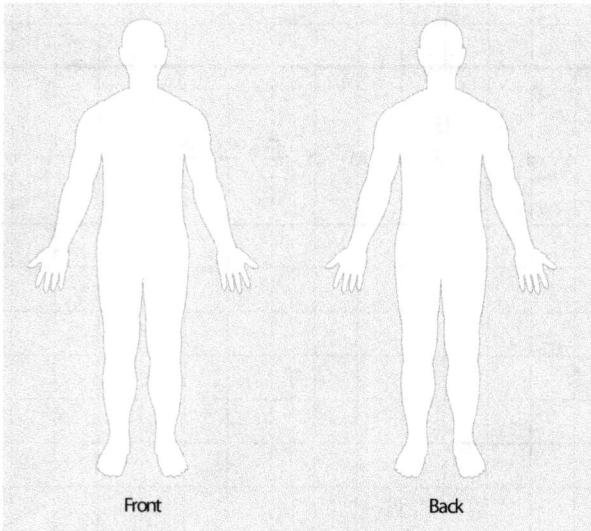

Front   Back

NON-DRUG THERAPIES
(other than prescription or other medicines)

_____

_____

ACTIVITIES/EXERCISE

_____

What was your average level of pain today?

0   1   2   3   4   5   6   7   8   9   10

Other than prescription medicine, did you do anything else today to relieve the pain? ____NO   ____YES:
(Note any that you used.)
____ Non-prescription drugs (e.g., acetaminophen, ibuprofen)
____ Herbal remedies
____ Hot or cold packs
____ Exercise
____ Changing position (such as lying down or elevating your legs)
____ Physical therapy
____ Massage
____ Acupuncture
____ Rest
____ Prayer, meditation, guided imagery
____ Relaxation technique (hypnosis, biofeedback)
____ Creative technique (art or music therapy)
____ Other (e.g., specific chiropractic manipulation, osteopathic treatments):

_____

Check any of these common side effects that you've noticed after taking your pain medicine:
____ Drowsiness, sleepiness
____ Nausea, vomiting, upset stomach
____ Constipation
____ Lack of appetite
____ Other (describe):

_____

Did you sleep through the night?   ____NO____YES

If not, how many times was your sleep disrupted? _____

How many hours did you sleep during the night? _____

COMMENTS AND MORE INFORMATION: Make notes for and about visits with your healthcare provider, side effects from treatments you may be experiencing, any problems you are having coping with your pain, and more about some of your previous answers or questions.

_____

_____

_____

6 DAILY BODY PAIN DIAGRAM

Mark each place on the diagram where you have had pain today by placing an 'X', circling the location, or shading the area .

Describe the type of pain:

Shooting	Deep
Tingling	Sharp
Numbness	Burning / Hot
Cold	Aching
Surface Pain	Gnawing / Biting
Stabbing	Electrical / Shocks
Dull	Other_____
Stinging	

COMMENTS AND MORE INFORMATION:

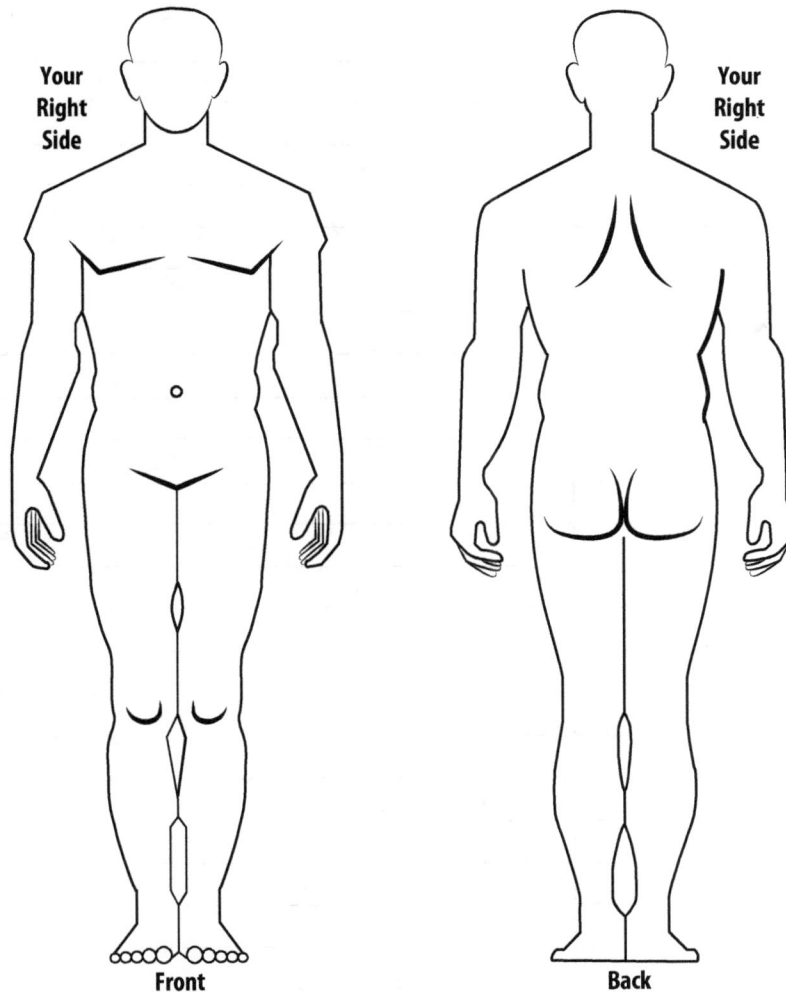

Your Right Side

Your Right Side

Front

Back

25

1 DAILY
TREATMENT PLAN

As you and your medical team develop new treatment plans, record your plan for the day including:
1.) New medications,
2.) Increases or decreases to medications,
3.) Exercises, physical therapy, or any other treatments,
4.) It will be especially helpful to record any side effects you experience as you add new treatments.
   This can help determine which types of treatments will work best for you.

Contact your care provider with any bad reactions or side effects to determine if you should discontinue the medication or treatment.

MEDICATION / TREATMENT	AMOUNT / TIME / COMMENTS

26

DAY_____ DATE_____ WEIGHT_____

INSTRUCTIONS:
1.) **Place an 'X'** on the chart below where the lines for the time of day and your level of pain meet.
2.) **Connect the points** on your DAILY PAIN CHART so your medical team can see when your status changed.
3.) **Refer to the EXAMPLES** in the front of this book for further direction.

2 DAILY PAIN CHART

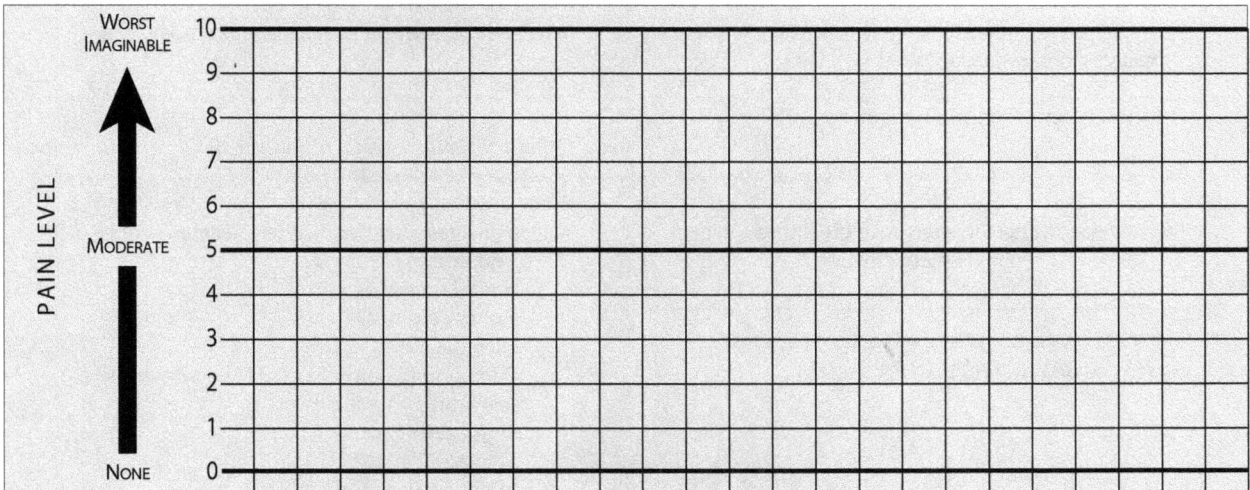

PAIN LEVEL

WORST IMAGINABLE

MODERATE

NONE

10
9
8
7
6
5
4
3
2
1
0

3 DAILY MEDICATION

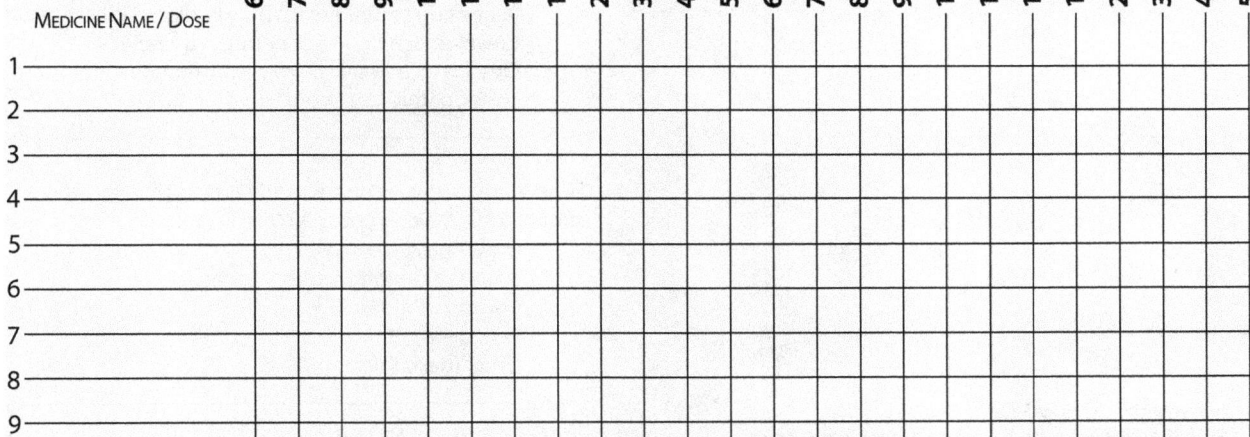

MEDICINE NAME / DOSE

6am 7 8 9 10 11 12pm 1 2 3 4 5 6pm 7 8 9 10 11 12am 1 2 3 4 5

1
2
3
4
5
6
7
8
9

4 DAILY PHYSIOLOGY

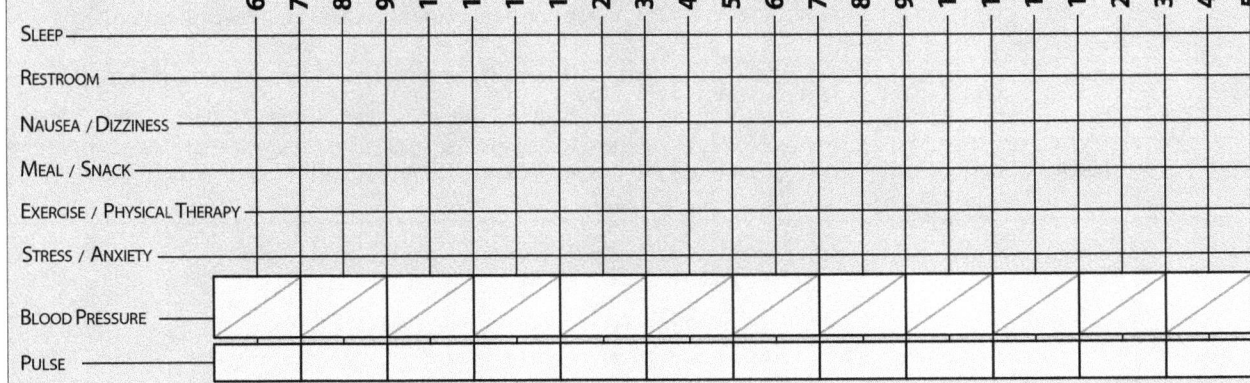

6am 7 8 9 10 11 12pm 1 2 3 4 5 6pm 7 8 9 10 11 12am 1 2 3 4 5

SLEEP

RESTROOM

NAUSEA / DIZZINESS

MEAL / SNACK

EXERCISE / PHYSICAL THERAPY

STRESS / ANXIETY

BLOOD PRESSURE

PULSE

26

5 DAILY
PAIN SUMMARY

Were there times during the day that you experienced unrelieved breakthrough pain? _____ NO _____ YES

How many times did this happen today?

1 2 3 4 5 6 7 8 9 10 more than 10

Did any specific activity start your breakthrough pain?
_____ NO _____ YES: What activities?

_____

Put an "X" on the body diagram to show each place you've had **BREAKTHROUGH PAIN** today.

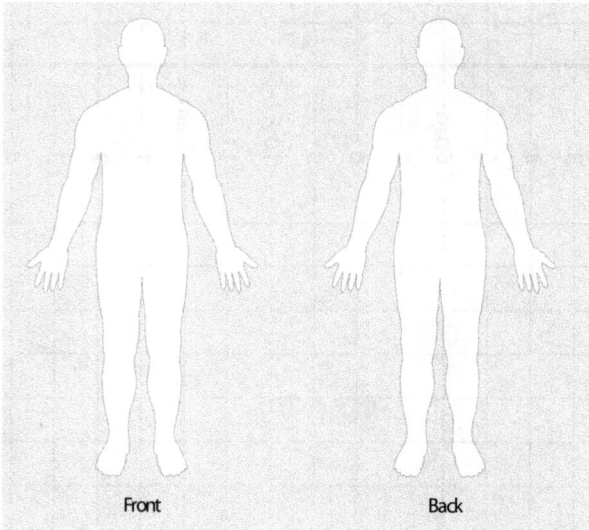

Front   Back

NON-DRUG THERAPIES
(other than prescription or other medicines)

_____

_____

ACTIVITIES/EXERCISE

_____

What was your average level of pain today?

0 1 2 3 4 5 6 7 8 9 10

Other than prescription medicine, did you do anything else today to relieve the pain? _____ NO _____ YES:
(Note any that you used.)
_____ Non-prescription drugs (e.g., acetaminophen, ibuprofen)
_____ Herbal remedies
_____ Hot or cold packs
_____ Exercise
_____ Changing position (such as lying down or elevating your legs)
_____ Physical therapy
_____ Massage
_____ Acupuncture
_____ Rest
_____ Prayer, meditation, guided imagery
_____ Relaxation technique (hypnosis, biofeedback)
_____ Creative technique (art or music therapy)
_____ Other (e.g., specific chiropractic manipulation, osteopathic treatments):

_____

Check any of these common side effects that you've noticed after taking your pain medicine:
_____ Drowsiness, sleepiness
_____ Nausea, vomiting, upset stomach
_____ Constipation
_____ Lack of appetite
_____ Other (describe):

_____

Did you sleep through the night? _____ NO _____ YES

If not, how many times was your sleep disrupted? _____

How many hours did you sleep during the night? _____

COMMENTS AND MORE INFORMATION: Make notes for and about visits with your healthcare provider, side effects from treatments you may be experiencing, any problems you are having coping with your pain, and more about some of your previous answers or questions.

_____

_____

_____

26

6 DAILY BODY PAIN DIAGRAM

Mark each place on the diagram where you have had pain today by placing an 'X', circling the location, or shading the area .

Describe the type of pain:

Shooting	Deep
Tingling	Sharp
Numbness	Burning / Hot
Cold	Aching
Surface Pain	Gnawing / Biting
Stabbing	Electrical / Shocks
Dull	Other_____
Stinging	

COMMENTS AND MORE INFORMATION:

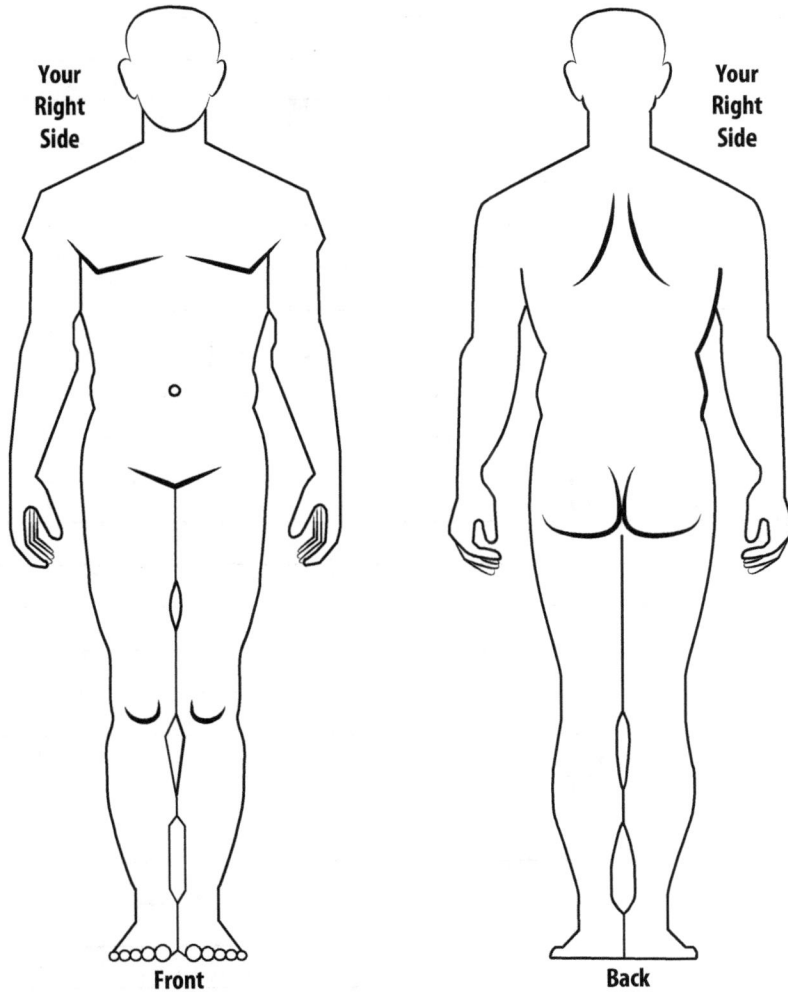

Your Right Side

Your Right Side

Front

Back

26

1 DAILY
TREATMENT PLAN

As you and your medical team develop new treatment plans, record your plan for the day including:
1.) New medications,
2.) Increases or decreases to medications,
3.) Exercises, physical therapy, or any other treatments,
4.) It will be especially helpful to record any side effects you experience as you add new treatments.
    This can help determine which types of treatments will work best for you.

Contact your care provider with any bad reactions or side effects to determine if you should discontinue the medication or treatment.

MEDICATION / TREATMENT	AMOUNT / TIME / COMMENTS

27

INSTRUCTIONS:

DAY_____ DATE_____ WEIGHT_____

1.) **Place an 'X'** on the chart below where the lines for the time of day and your level of pain meet.
2.) **Connect the points** on your DAILY PAIN CHART so your medical team can see when your status changed.
3.) **Refer to the EXAMPLES** in the front of this book for further direction.

2 DAILY PAIN CHART

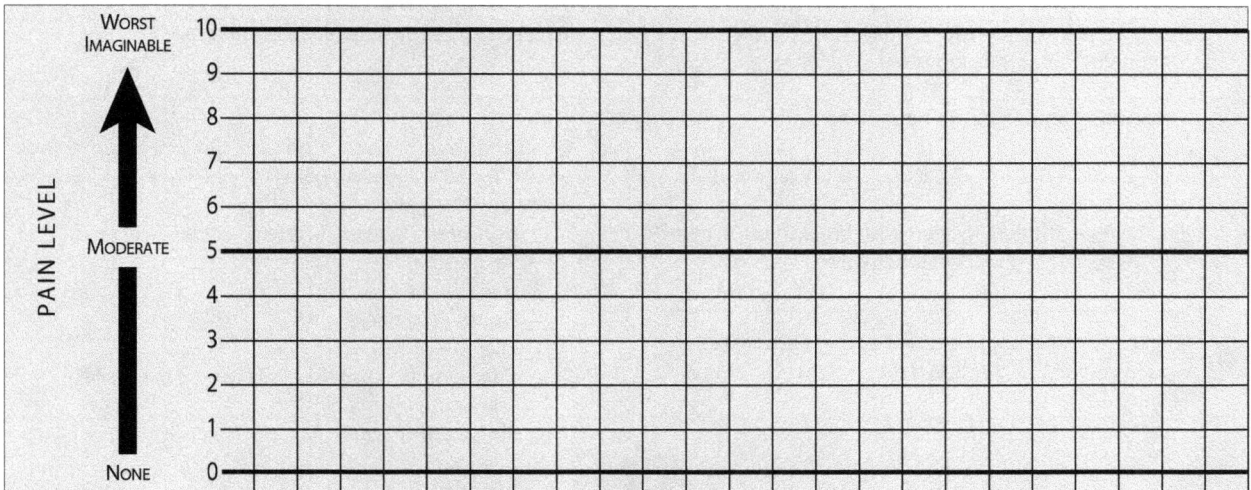

PAIN LEVEL

WORST IMAGINABLE — 10

9

8

7

6

MODERATE — 5

4

3

2

1

NONE — 0

3 DAILY MEDICATION

MEDICINE NAME / DOSE

	6am	7	8	9	10	11	12pm	1	2	3	4	5	6pm	7	8	9	10	11	12am	1	2	3	4	5
1																								
2																								
3																								
4																								
5																								
6																								
7																								
8																								
9																								

4 DAILY PHYSIOLOGY

	6am	7	8	9	10	11	12pm	1	2	3	4	5	6pm	7	8	9	10	11	12am	1	2	3	4	5
SLEEP																								
RESTROOM																								
NAUSEA / DIZZINESS																								
MEAL / SNACK																								
EXERCISE / PHYSICAL THERAPY																								
STRESS / ANXIETY																								
BLOOD PRESSURE																								
PULSE																								

27

5 DAILY
PAIN SUMMARY

Were there times during the day that you experienced unrelieved breakthrough pain? _____NO _____YES

How many times did this happen today?

    1 2 3 4 5 6 7 8 9 10 more than 10

Did any specific activity start your breakthrough pain? _____NO _____YES: What activities?

_____

Put an "X" on the body diagram to show each place you've had **BREAKTHROUGH PAIN** today.

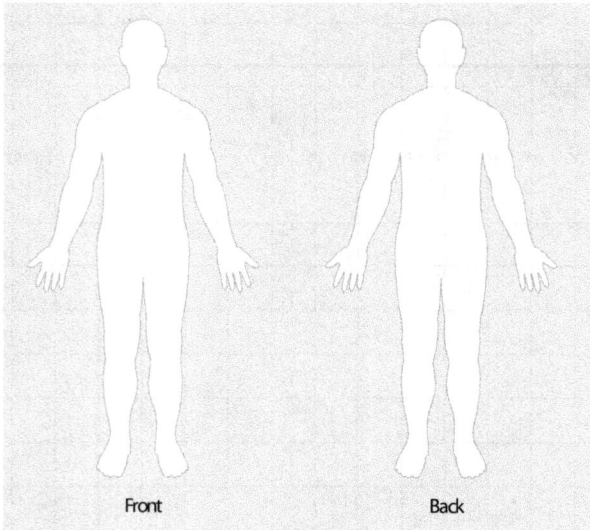

Front   Back

NON-DRUG THERAPIES
(other than prescription or other medicines)

_____

_____

ACTIVITIES/EXERCISE

_____

What was your average level of pain today?

    0 1 2 3 4 5 6 7 8 9 10

Other than prescription medicine, did you do anything else today to relieve the pain? _____NO _____YES: (Note any that you used.)
_____ Non-prescription drugs (e.g., acetaminophen, ibuprofen)
_____ Herbal remedies
_____ Hot or cold packs
_____ Exercise
_____ Changing position (such as lying down or elevating your legs)
_____ Physical therapy
_____ Massage
_____ Acupuncture
_____ Rest
_____ Prayer, meditation, guided imagery
_____ Relaxation technique (hypnosis, biofeedback)
_____ Creative technique (art or music therapy)
_____ Other (e.g., specific chiropractic manipulation, osteopathic treatments):

_____

Check any of these common side effects that you've noticed after taking your pain medicine:
_____ Drowsiness, sleepiness
_____ Nausea, vomiting, upset stomach
_____ Constipation
_____ Lack of appetite
_____ Other (describe):

_____

Did you sleep through the night? _____NO_____YES

If not, how many times was your sleep disrupted? _____

How many hours did you sleep during the night? _____

COMMENTS AND MORE INFORMATION: Make notes for and about visits with your healthcare provider, side effects from treatments you may be experiencing, any problems you are having coping with your pain, and more about some of your previous answers or questions.

_____

_____

_____

27

6 DAILY BODY PAIN DIAGRAM

Mark each place on the diagram where you have had pain today by placing an 'X', circling the location, or shading the area .

Describe the type of pain:

Shooting
Tingling
Numbness
Cold
Surface Pain
Stabbing
Dull
Stinging

Deep
Sharp
Burning / Hot
Aching
Gnawing / Biting
Electrical / Shocks
Other_____

COMMENTS AND MORE INFORMATION:

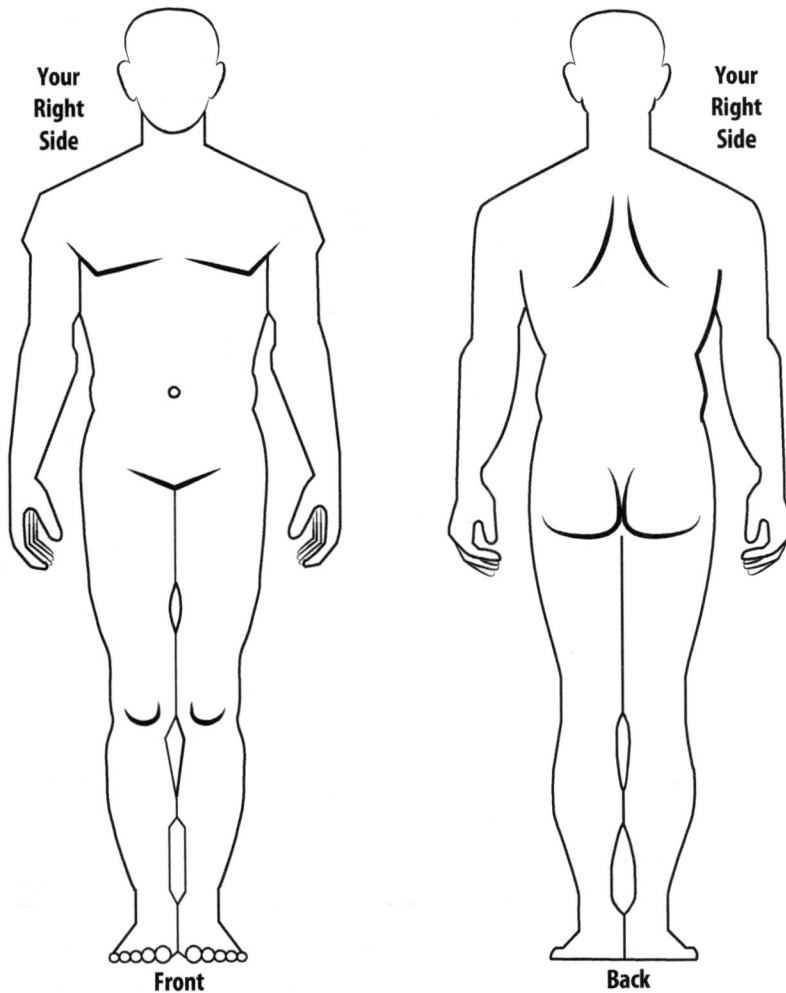

Your Right Side

Your Right Side

Front

Back

27

1 DAILY
TREATMENT PLAN

As you and your medical team develop new treatment plans, record your plan for the day including:

1.) New medications,
2.) Increases or decreases to medications,
3.) Exercises, physical therapy, or any other treatments,
4.) It will be especially helpful to record any side effects you experience as you add new treatments. This can help determine which types of treatments will work best for you.

Contact your care provider with any bad reactions or side effects to determine if you should discontinue the medication or treatment.

MEDICATION / TREATMENT	AMOUNT / TIME / COMMENTS

28

DAY_____ DATE_____ WEIGHT_____

INSTRUCTIONS:
1.) **Place an 'X'** on the chart below where the lines for the time of day and your level of pain meet.
2.) **Connect the points** on your DAILY PAIN CHART so your medical team can see when your status changed.
3.) **Refer to the EXAMPLES** in the front of this book for further direction.

2 DAILY PAIN CHART

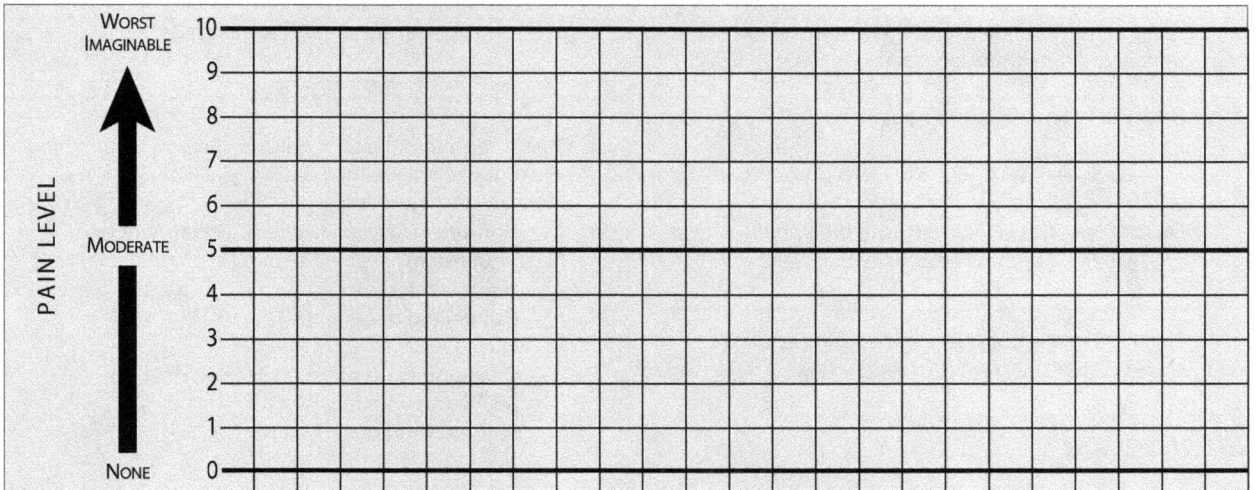

PAIN LEVEL		
WORST IMAGINABLE	10	
	9	
	8	
	7	
	6	
MODERATE	5	
	4	
	3	
	2	
	1	
NONE	0	

3 DAILY MEDICATION

MEDICINE NAME / DOSE

Times: 6am 7 8 9 10 11 12pm 1 2 3 4 5 6pm 7 8 9 10 11 12am 1 2 3 4 5

1
2
3
4
5
6
7
8
9

4 DAILY PHYSIOLOGY

Times: 6am 7 8 9 10 11 12pm 1 2 3 4 5 6pm 7 8 9 10 11 12am 1 2 3 4 5

SLEEP
RESTROOM
NAUSEA / DIZZINESS
MEAL / SNACK
EXERCISE / PHYSICAL THERAPY
STRESS / ANXIETY
BLOOD PRESSURE
PULSE

28

5 DAILY
PAIN SUMMARY

Were there times during the day that you experienced unrelieved breakthrough pain? _____NO _____YES

How many times did this happen today?

1 2 3 4 5 6 7 8 9 10 more than 10

Did any specific activity start your breakthrough pain? _____NO _____YES: What activities?

_____

Put an "X" on the body diagram to show each place you've had *BREAKTHROUGH PAIN* today.

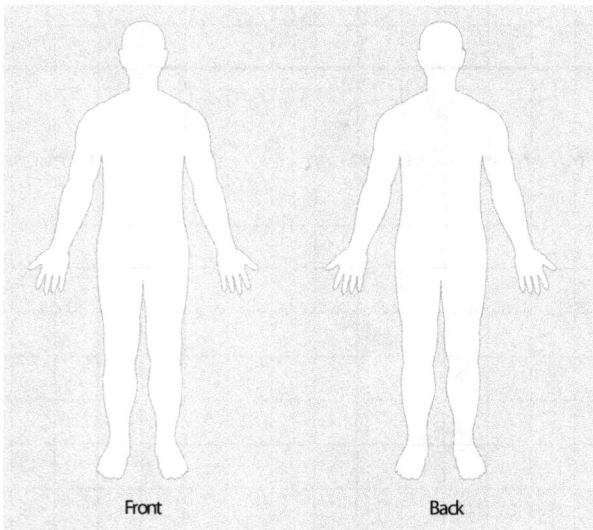

Front   Back

NON-DRUG THERAPIES
(other than prescription or other medicines)

_____

_____

ACTIVITIES/EXERCISE

_____

_____

What was your average level of pain today?

0   1   2   3   4   5   6   7   8   9   10

Other than prescription medicine, did you do anything else today to relieve the pain? _____NO _____YES:
(Note any that you used.)
_____ Non-prescription drugs (e.g., acetaminophen, ibuprofen)
_____ Herbal remedies
_____ Hot or cold packs
_____ Exercise
_____ Changing position (such as lying down or elevating your legs)
_____ Physical therapy
_____ Massage
_____ Acupuncture
_____ Rest
_____ Prayer, meditation, guided imagery
_____ Relaxation technique (hypnosis, biofeedback)
_____ Creative technique (art or music therapy)
_____ Other (e.g., specific chiropractic manipulation, osteopathic treatments):

_____

Check any of these common side effects that you've noticed after taking your pain medicine:
_____ Drowsiness, sleepiness
_____ Nausea, vomiting, upset stomach
_____ Constipation
_____ Lack of appetite
_____ Other (describe):

_____

Did you sleep through the night? _____NO_____YES

If not, how many times was your sleep disrupted? _____

How many hours did you sleep during the night? _____

COMMENTS AND MORE INFORMATION: Make notes for and about visits with your healthcare provider, side effects from treatments you may be experiencing, any problems you are having coping with your pain, and more about some of your previous answers or questions.

_____

_____

_____

28

6 DAILY BODY PAIN DIAGRAM

Mark each place on the diagram where you have had pain today by placing an 'X', circling the location, or shading the area .

Describe the type of pain:

Shooting	Deep
Tingling	Sharp
Numbness	Burning / Hot
Cold	Aching
Surface Pain	Gnawing / Biting
Stabbing	Electrical / Shocks
Dull	Other_____
Stinging	

COMMENTS AND MORE INFORMATION:

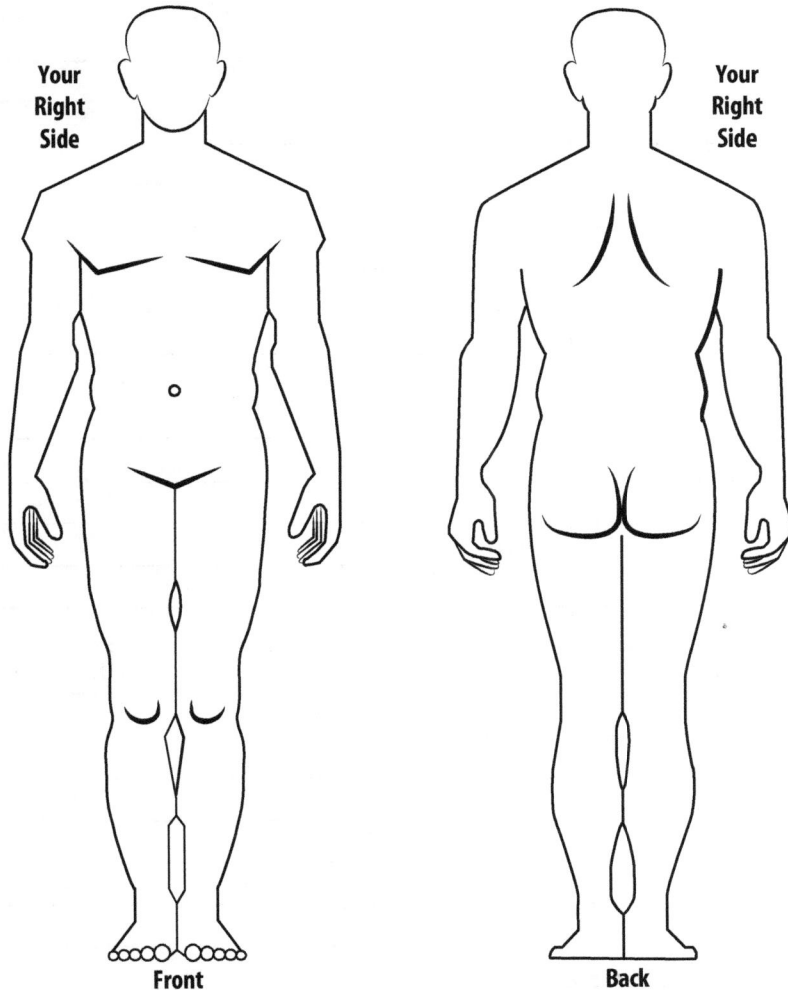

Your
Right
Side

Your
Right
Side

Front

Back

28

1 DAILY
TREATMENT PLAN

29

As you and your medical team develop new treatment plans, record your plan for the day including:
1.) New medications,
2.) Increases or decreases to medications,
3.) Exercises, physical therapy, or any other treatments,
4.) It will be especially helpful to record any side effects you experience as you add new treatments.
    This can help determine which types of treatments will work best for you.

Contact your care provider with any bad reactions or side effects to determine if you should discontinue the medication or treatment.

MEDICATION / TREATMENT	AMOUNT / TIME / COMMENTS

INSTRUCTIONS:
1.) **Place an 'X'** on the chart below where the lines for the time of day and your level of pain meet.
2.) **Connect the points** on your DAILY PAIN CHART so your medical team can see when your status changed.
3.) **Refer to the EXAMPLES** in the front of this book for further direction.

DAY_____ DATE_____ WEIGHT_____

29

2 DAILY PAIN CHART

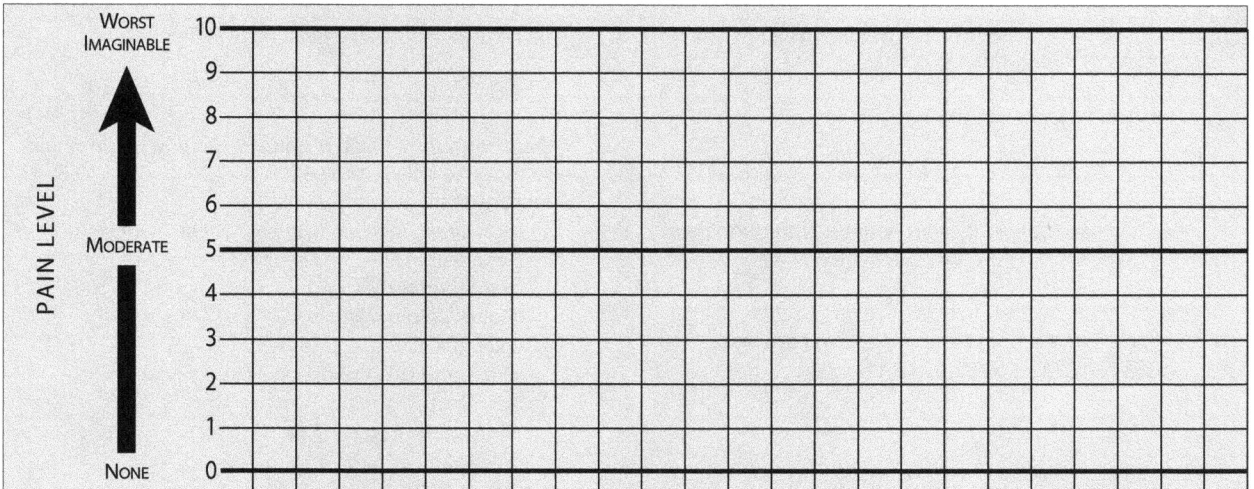

PAIN LEVEL

WORST IMAGINABLE	10
	9
	8
	7
	6
MODERATE	5
	4
	3
	2
	1
NONE	0

3 DAILY MEDICATION

MEDICINE NAME / DOSE

6am 7 8 9 10 11 12pm 1 2 3 4 5 6pm 7 8 9 10 11 12am 1 2 3 4 5

1
2
3
4
5
6
7
8
9

4 DAILY PHYSIOLOGY

6am 7 8 9 10 11 12pm 1 2 3 4 5 6pm 7 8 9 10 11 12am 1 2 3 4 5

SLEEP
RESTROOM
NAUSEA / DIZZINESS
MEAL / SNACK
EXERCISE / PHYSICAL THERAPY
STRESS / ANXIETY
BLOOD PRESSURE
PULSE

5 DAILY
PAIN SUMMARY

Were there times during the day that you experienced unrelieved breakthrough pain? ____NO ____YES

How many times did this happen today?

1 2 3 4 5 6 7 8 9 10 more than 10

Did any specific activity start your breakthrough pain? ____NO ____YES: What activities?

_____

Put an "X" on the body diagram to show each place you've had **BREAKTHROUGH PAIN** today.

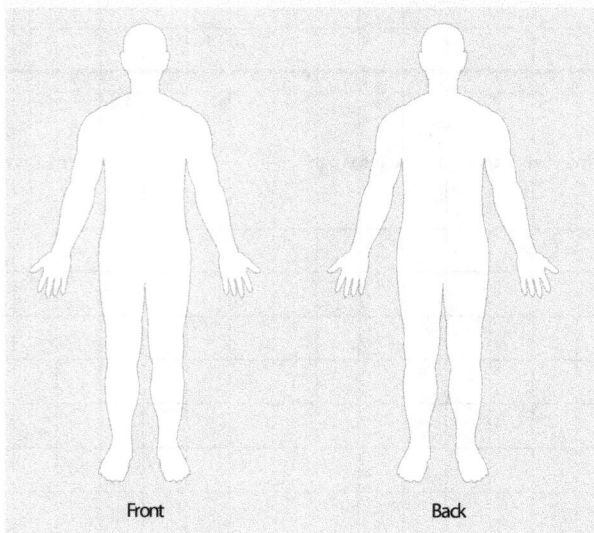

Front   Back

NON-DRUG THERAPIES
(other than prescription or other medicines)

_____

_____

ACTIVITIES/EXERCISE

_____

What was your average level of pain today?

0   1   2   3   4   5   6   7   8   9   10

Other than prescription medicine, did you do anything else today to relieve the pain? ____NO ____YES:
(Note any that you used.)
____ Non-prescription drugs (e.g., acetaminophen, ibuprofen)
____ Herbal remedies
____ Hot or cold packs
____ Exercise
____ Changing position (such as lying down or elevating your legs)
____ Physical therapy
____ Massage
____ Acupuncture
____ Rest
____ Prayer, meditation, guided imagery
____ Relaxation technique (hypnosis, biofeedback)
____ Creative technique (art or music therapy)
____ Other (e.g., specific chiropractic manipulation, osteopathic treatments):

_____

Check any of these common side effects that you've noticed after taking your pain medicine:
____ Drowsiness, sleepiness
____ Nausea, vomiting, upset stomach
____ Constipation
____ Lack of appetite
____ Other (describe):

_____

Did you sleep through the night? ____NO____YES

If not, how many times was your sleep disrupted? _____

How many hours did you sleep during the night? _____

COMMENTS AND MORE INFORMATION: Make notes for and about visits with your healthcare provider, side effects from treatments you may be experiencing, any problems you are having coping with your pain, and more about some of your previous answers or questions.

_____

_____

_____

6 DAILY BODY PAIN DIAGRAM

Mark each place on the diagram where you have had pain today by placing an 'X', circling the location, or shading the area .

Describe the type of pain:

Shooting	Deep
Tingling	Sharp
Numbness	Burning / Hot
Cold	Aching
Surface Pain	Gnawing / Biting
Stabbing	Electrical / Shocks
Dull	Other_____
Stinging	

COMMENTS AND MORE INFORMATION:

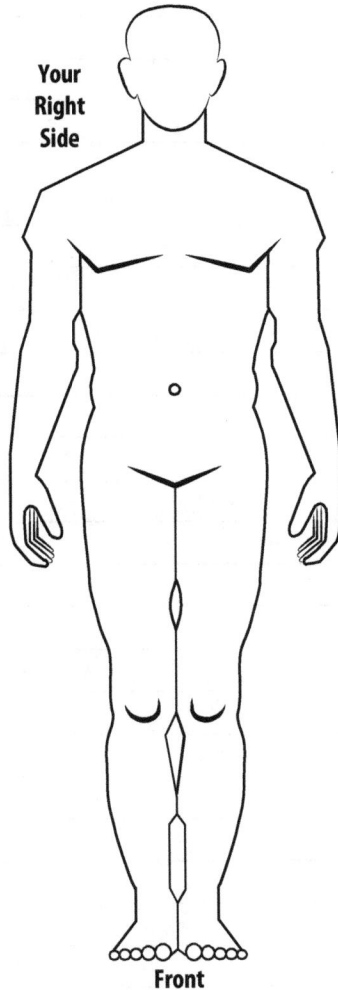

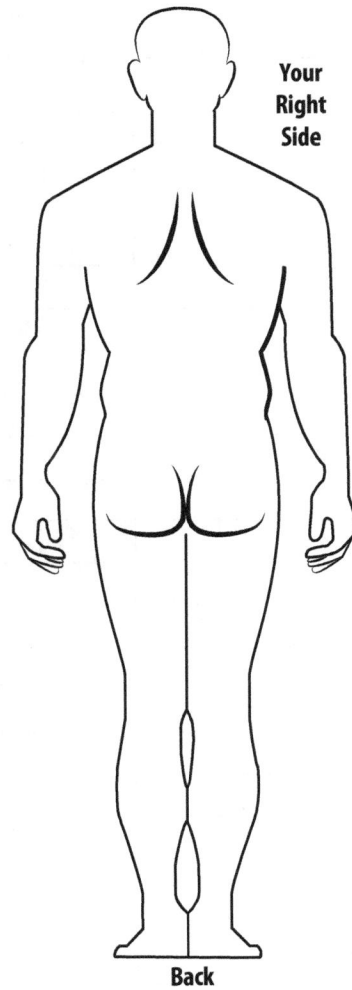

Your Right Side

Front

Your Right Side

Back

1 DAILY
TREATMENT PLAN

As you and your medical team develop new treatment plans, record your plan for the day including:
1.) New medications,
2.) Increases or decreases to medications,
3.) Exercises, physical therapy, or any other treatments,
4.) It will be especially helpful to record any side effects you experience as you add new treatments. This can help determine which types of treatments will work best for you.

Contact your care provider with any bad reactions or side effects to determine if you should discontinue the medication or treatment.

30

MEDICATION / TREATMENT	AMOUNT / TIME / COMMENTS

DAY_____ DATE_____ WEIGHT_____

INSTRUCTIONS:
1.) **Place an 'X'** on the chart below where the lines for the time of day and your level of pain meet.
2.) **Connect the points** on your DAILY PAIN CHART so your medical team can see when your status changed.
3.) **Refer to the EXAMPLES** in the front of this book for further direction.

2 DAILY PAIN CHART

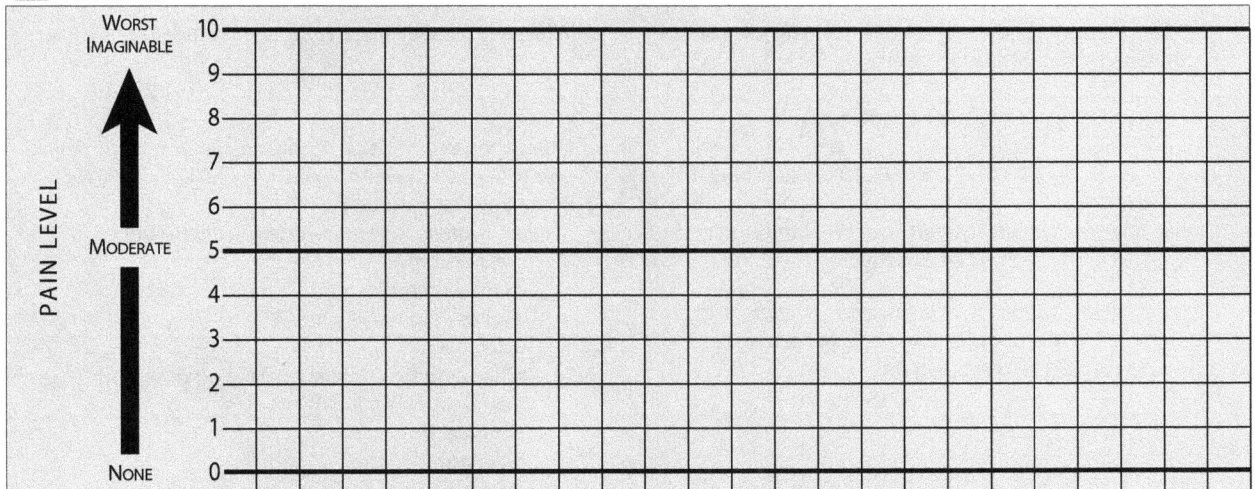

PAIN LEVEL

WORST IMAGINABLE — 10
9
8
7
6
MODERATE — 5
4
3
2
1
NONE — 0

3 DAILY MEDICATION

MEDICINE NAME / DOSE

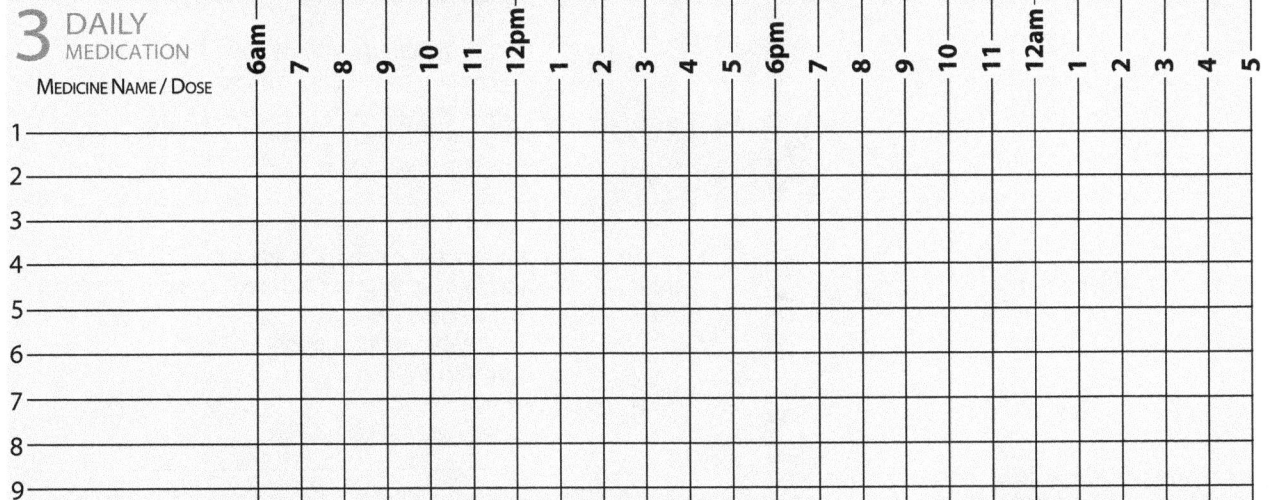

Times: 6am, 7, 8, 9, 10, 11, 12pm, 1, 2, 3, 4, 5, 6pm, 7, 8, 9, 10, 11, 12am, 1, 2, 3, 4, 5

1
2
3
4
5
6
7
8
9

4 DAILY PHYSIOLOGY

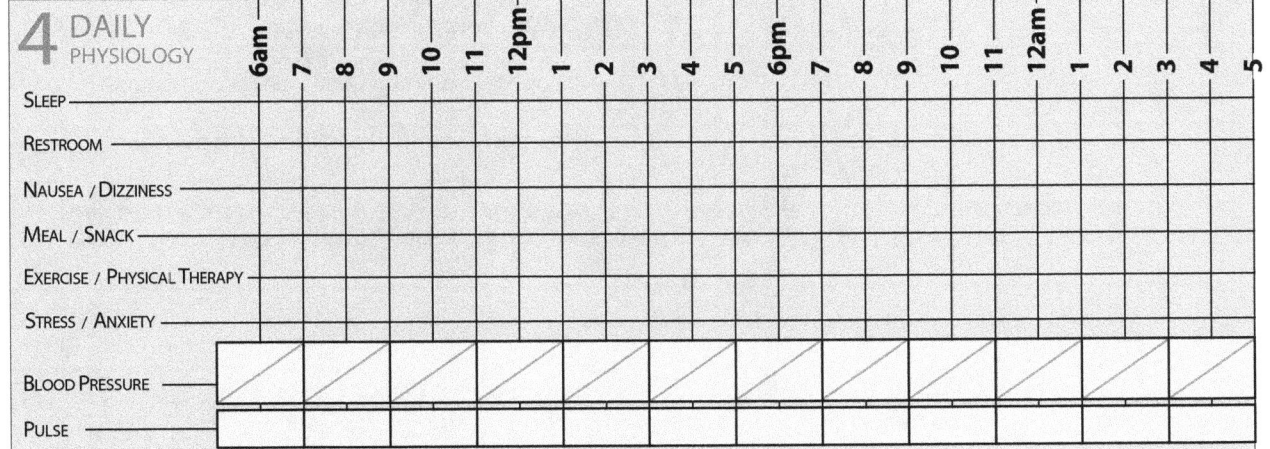

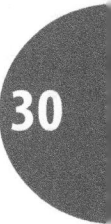

Times: 6am, 7, 8, 9, 10, 11, 12pm, 1, 2, 3, 4, 5, 6pm, 7, 8, 9, 10, 11, 12am, 1, 2, 3, 4, 5

SLEEP
RESTROOM
NAUSEA / DIZZINESS
MEAL / SNACK
EXERCISE / PHYSICAL THERAPY
STRESS / ANXIETY
BLOOD PRESSURE
PULSE

30

5 DAILY
PAIN SUMMARY

Were there times during the day that you experienced unrelieved breakthrough pain? _____NO _____YES

How many times did this happen today?

   1 2 3 4 5 6 7 8 9 10 more than 10

Did any specific activity start your breakthrough pain? _____NO _____YES: What activities?

_____

Put an "X" on the body diagram to show each place you've had **BREAKTHROUGH PAIN** today.

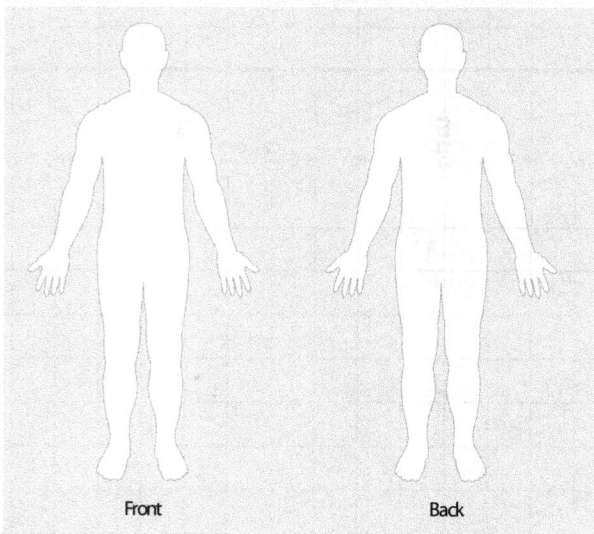

Front   Back

NON-DRUG THERAPIES
(other than prescription or other medicines)

_____

_____

ACTIVITIES/EXERCISE

_____

_____

What was your average level of pain today?

   0 1 2 3 4 5 6 7 8 9 10

Other than prescription medicine, did you do anything else today to relieve the pain? _____NO _____YES: (Note any that you used.)
_____ Non-prescription drugs (e.g., acetaminophen, ibuprofen)
_____ Herbal remedies
_____ Hot or cold packs
_____ Exercise
_____ Changing position (such as lying down or elevating your legs)
_____ Physical therapy
_____ Massage
_____ Acupuncture
_____ Rest
_____ Prayer, meditation, guided imagery
_____ Relaxation technique (hypnosis, biofeedback)
_____ Creative technique (art or music therapy)
_____ Other (e.g., specific chiropractic manipulation, osteopathic treatments):

_____

Check any of these common side effects that you've noticed after taking your pain medicine:
_____ Drowsiness, sleepiness
_____ Nausea, vomiting, upset stomach
_____ Constipation
_____ Lack of appetite
_____ Other (describe):

_____

Did you sleep through the night? _____NO_____YES

If not, how many times was your sleep disrupted? _____

How many hours did you sleep during the night? _____

COMMENTS AND MORE INFORMATION: Make notes for and about visits with your healthcare provider, side effects from treatments you may be experiencing, any problems you are having coping with your pain, and more about some of your previous answers or questions.

_____

_____

30

6 DAILY BODY PAIN DIAGRAM

Mark each place on the diagram where you have had pain today by placing an 'X', circling the location, or shading the area.

Describe the type of pain:

Shooting   Deep
Tingling   Sharp
Numbness   Burning / Hot
Cold   Aching
Surface Pain   Gnawing / Biting
Stabbing   Electrical / Shocks
Dull   Other_____
Stinging

COMMENTS AND MORE INFORMATION:

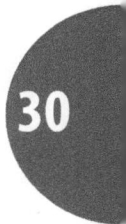

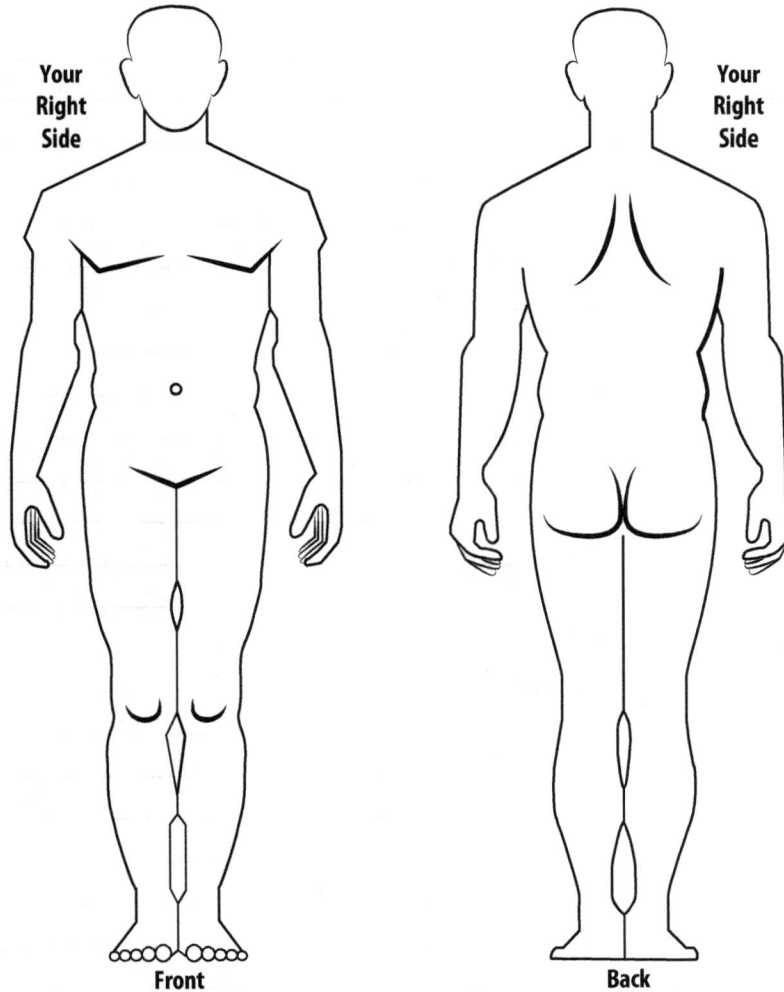

30

Your Right Side

Your Right Side

Front

Back

1 DAILY
TREATMENT PLAN

As you and your medical team develop new treatment plans, record your plan for the day including:
1.) New medications,
2.) Increases or decreases to medications,
3.) Exercises, physical therapy, or any other treatments,
4.) It will be especially helpful to record any side effects you experience as you add new treatments.
   This can help determine which types of treatments will work best for you.

Contact your care provider with any bad reactions or side effects to determine if you should discontinue
the medication or treatment.

MEDICATION / TREATMENT	AMOUNT / TIME / COMMENTS

31

INSTRUCTIONS:

DAY_____ DATE_____ WEIGHT_____

1.) **Place an 'X'** on the chart below where the lines for the time of day and your level of pain meet.
2.) **Connect the points** on your DAILY PAIN CHART so your medical team can see when your status changed.
3.) **Refer to the EXAMPLES** in the front of this book for further direction.

2 DAILY PAIN CHART

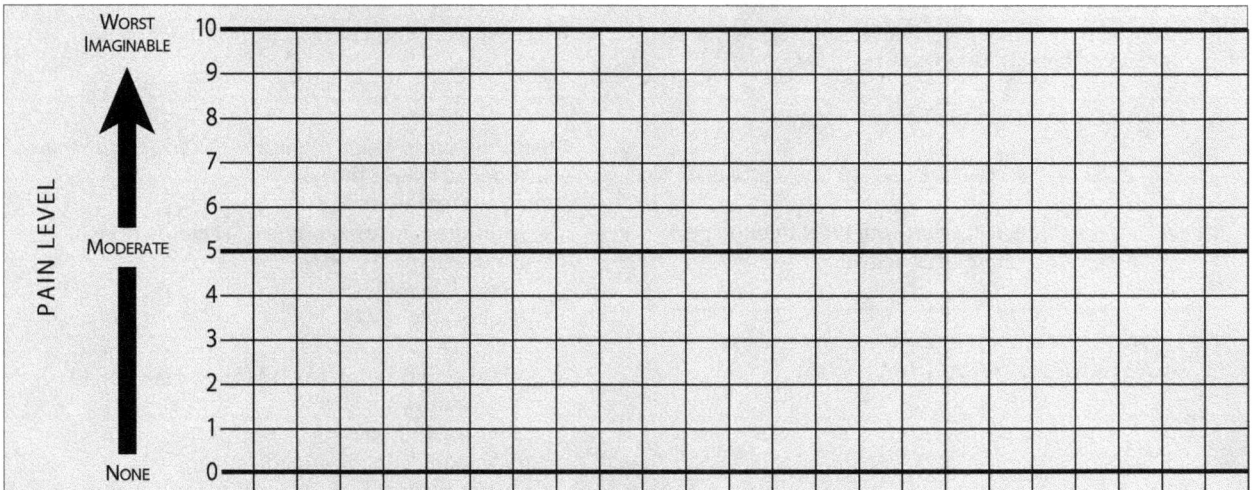

PAIN LEVEL

WORST IMAGINABLE	10
	9
	8
	7
	6
MODERATE	5
	4
	3
	2
	1
NONE	0

3 DAILY MEDICATION

MEDICINE NAME / DOSE

Times: 6am, 7, 8, 9, 10, 11, 12pm, 1, 2, 3, 4, 5, 6pm, 7, 8, 9, 10, 11, 12am, 1, 2, 3, 4, 5

1
2
3
4
5
6
7
8
9

4 DAILY PHYSIOLOGY

Times: 6am, 7, 8, 9, 10, 11, 12pm, 1, 2, 3, 4, 5, 6pm, 7, 8, 9, 10, 11, 12am, 1, 2, 3, 4, 5

SLEEP
RESTROOM
NAUSEA / DIZZINESS
MEAL / SNACK
EXERCISE / PHYSICAL THERAPY
STRESS / ANXIETY
BLOOD PRESSURE
PULSE

31

5 DAILY
PAIN SUMMARY

Were there times during the day that you experienced unrelieved breakthrough pain? ____NO ____YES

How many times did this happen today?

  1 2 3 4 5 6 7 8 9 10 more than 10

Did any specific activity start your breakthrough pain? ____NO ____YES: What activities?

_____

Put an "X" on the body diagram to show each place you've had **BREAKTHROUGH PAIN** today.

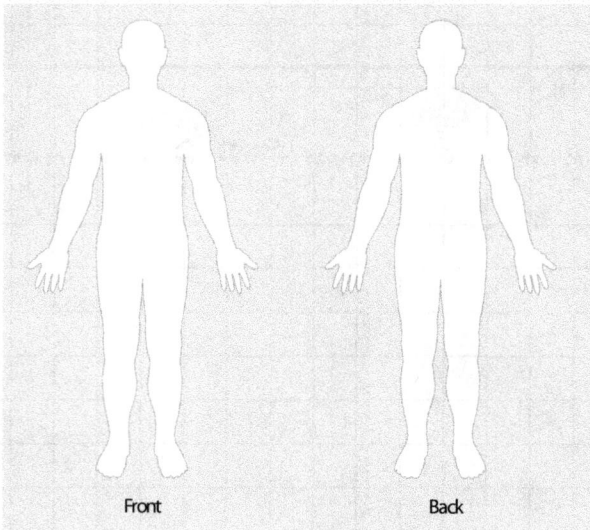

Front   Back

NON-DRUG THERAPIES
(other than prescription or other medicines)

_____

_____

ACTIVITIES/EXERCISE

_____

What was your average level of pain today?

  0 1 2 3 4 5 6 7 8 9 10

Other than prescription medicine, did you do anything else today to relieve the pain? ____NO ____YES: (Note any that you used.)
____ Non-prescription drugs (e.g., acetaminophen, ibuprofen)
____ Herbal remedies
____ Hot or cold packs
____ Exercise
____ Changing position (such as lying down or elevating your legs)
____ Physical therapy
____ Massage
____ Acupuncture
____ Rest
____ Prayer, meditation, guided imagery
____ Relaxation technique (hypnosis, biofeedback)
____ Creative technique (art or music therapy)
____ Other (e.g., specific chiropractic manipulation, osteopathic treatments):

_____

Check any of these common side effects that you've noticed after taking your pain medicine:
____ Drowsiness, sleepiness
____ Nausea, vomiting, upset stomach
____ Constipation
____ Lack of appetite
____ Other (describe):

_____

Did you sleep through the night? ____NO____YES

If not, how many times was your sleep disrupted? _____

How many hours did you sleep during the night? _____

COMMENTS AND MORE INFORMATION: Make notes for and about visits with your healthcare provider, side effects from treatments you may be experiencing, any problems you are having coping with your pain, and more about some of your previous answers or questions.

_____

_____

_____

6 DAILY BODY PAIN DIAGRAM

Mark each place on the diagram where you have had pain today by placing an 'X', circling the location, or shading the area .

Describe the type of pain:

Shooting	Deep
Tingling	Sharp
Numbness	Burning / Hot
Cold	Aching
Surface Pain	Gnawing / Biting
Stabbing	Electrical / Shocks
Dull	Other_____
Stinging	

COMMENTS AND MORE INFORMATION:

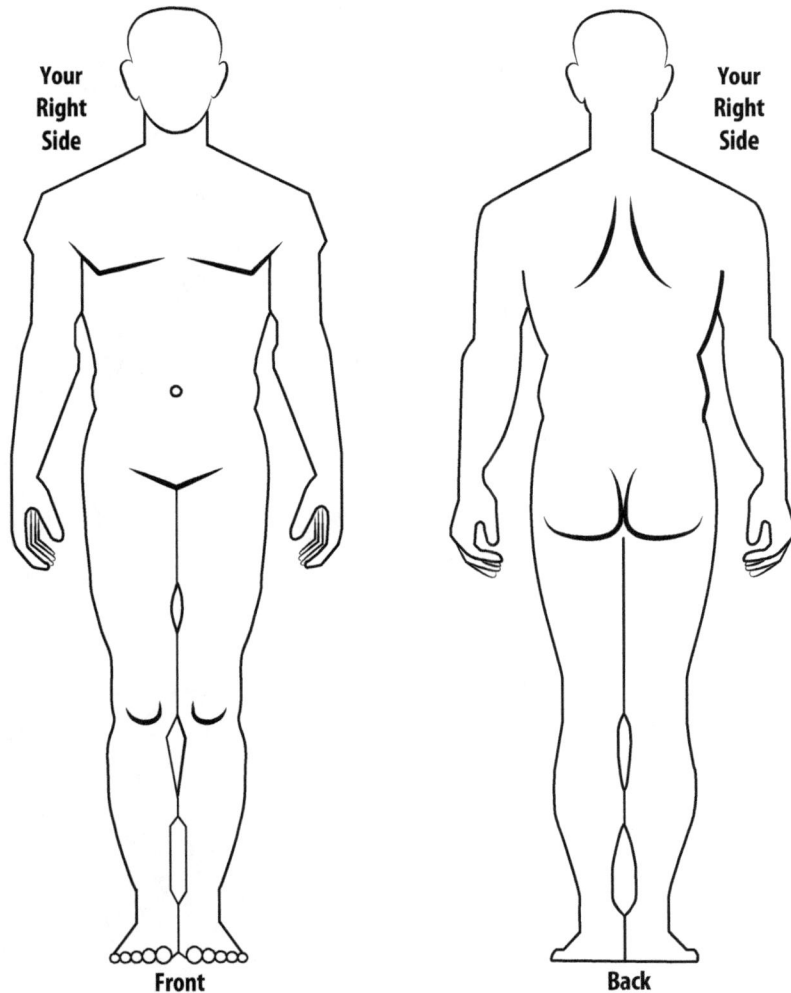

31

Your Right Side

Your Right Side

Front

Back

www.ingramcontent.com/pod-product-compliance
Lightning Source LLC
Chambersburg PA
CBHW080614270326
41928CB00016B/3059